Praise for Kaelin Tuell Poulin & *BIG FAT LIES*

Andrea Carter

I needed Kaelin, this program. She saved my life, gave me confidence, strength, and has made me a better mom. This program is a lifestyle change and I've never felt better. I have a long ways to go but because of the LadyBoss program I know I can do this and I have my identity back.

Nikki Nelson

6 MONTHS—That is all it has taken to change my life forever. I was feeling better just weeks into the program. This program and Kaelin literally saved my life. Don't give up ladies! Trust the process, and you'll see progress.

Angeline Wiersema

I followed Kaelin for months before I finally decided that the LadyBoss program was exactly what I needed in my life. I've tried everything for weight-loss—from pills, to wraps, diets, working out, etc. You name it and I've probably tried it. It wasn't until watching Kaelin that I finally understood what I was missing. I didn't understand that it's not about weight-loss or even "dieting." It's about changing your lifestyle and loving yourself for who you already are. And that's when I decided that this program was for me.

Jennifer Webb

While recovering from my surgeries, I came across one of Kaelin's Facebook videos and became so intrigued by how real and honest she was. I did some more "research" and started to watch Kaelin's YouTube videos and LOVED everything about what she had to offer! It sounds funny, but I felt like she was talking directly to me on certain levels!

I'm SO HAPPY to say I've lost 20 lbs! YES!!!!!!!!! This is ALL THANKS to Kaelin and the amazing LadyBoss program! I've learned to ALWAYS make myself a priority and that includes working out every day and eating healthy!

Alexandria Blue

Although people can see and comment on the weight I've lost, I think the biggest thing I've taken away from this program honestly is mental. I'm so much happier with who I am now. I have Kaelin to thank for that. I feel like a new woman, a stronger, happier, more positive, adventurous one. I'm never going back.

Brittany Karas

LadyBoss has what a lot of programs are missing. There is constant support from a group of great ladies, an encouraging leader who tells it how it is, and is present in your journey and this program is COMPLETE. It isn't just workout, just diet or just support. It's all three and more. This program has not only changed my body and mindset but my whole lifestyle. I have gained my smile back and my confidence. I have gained the desire to do the old things I used to do that make me happy. I have gained the desire to go spend time with friends. I have gained the desire to eat healthy and be active. I have gained the desire to show my niece and nephew the way to live a healthy life. LadyBoss has changed my life. I have Kaelin to thank for that. LadyBoss for life.

Kaylenn Gosman

I have tried it all from crash diets, diet pills, detox teas, weight-loss shakes — you name it, I've done it. But those were all temporary for me. One day I was laying in bed upset about my weight, which was an everyday thing, and saw Kaelin had posted a live feed. I had never heard of her or her progress or program before so I watched her 45 minute feed and ended up buying the lifetime deal with LadyBoss. With this program I feel like a completely different person. I will never forget the day I randomly met Kaelin in Louisville at the gym and the encouragement she gave me. She cares about her LadyBosses and their progress! I love this lifetime program!!!

Morgan Deardorff

Since starting this journey I have not only lost 5 pounds and 1% body fat but have also lost a jean size! Along with that I have gained the most confidence I've ever had in my own skin. I walk into the gym with my head held high and know I will crush my workout because I know exactly what I'm going to do ahead of time. I have already come so far in 6 weeks and can't wait to see how much farther I can go! I get married next April and plan to blow everyone away! Thank you, Kaelin for creating such an amazing and easy to follow program, you have changed my life for the better!

Tasha Ford

When I saw and read the story on LadyBoss I was sold! I have a meal plan! Workouts! And motivating and inspirational ladies to help me on my journey every day! I have lost 7lbs, I'm feeling better then ever and motivated to reach my goal. Thank you, Kaelin for pushing me everyday! I love being part of something so wonderful.

Braylen Unser

If it wasn't for Kaelin and the LadyBoss app, I don't think I would be where I am now because this is the longest I've ever stuck to a program or routine. The Facebook group truly does give everyone the extra push they need and allow for accountability. I am so happy for this safe place where I can post anything about my fitness journey and not be embarrassed. Many women need that and it's so awesome that it is now accessible! I am so excited for more things to come! Thank you, Kaelin.

Macil Melton

I feel amazing, and my BF/BMI % has already dropped. I have more confidence after joining the LadyBoss movement, I feel stronger both physically and emotionally and I just can't thank Kaelin or the awesome LadyBosses in the group enough!!!

Katie Peoe

This is the first time in my entire life I have gotten the food thing and the gym thing going at the same time. I have incredible amounts of energy and my focus has not wavered one bit. I love being a LadyBoss and am excited to show my daughter how a LadyBoss does it! Thank you, Kaelin.

Hannah Turner

I have tried everything I can to lose weight but I begin to lose motivation until now. I have eaten much healthier and worked out more then ever and I love it! It has now become a lifestyle change. We want to have kids soon and I need to be the best mom physically for them so they can grow up in a healthy home! Thank you for what you do and for being an inspiration to, not only me but, all these amazing LadyBoss women!

Michelle Brown

I was watching a video Kaelin made and something just clicked one day! If I brush my teeth every day, I need to go to the gym! It's a healthy habit! So I've finally made the gym a habit and love it! I am more confident, very happy with my life and myself right now! Kaelin and this group of wonderful women has changed my life! My outlook on life has changed and I'm in control of myself! I will be working toward becoming as fit and healthy I can be for my wedding on April 1, 2017!

Serene Kae

What I have learned from LadyBoss Ultimate Transformation Academy is how to refocus my purpose of why, what, and when I eat! I am constantly shifting my filter to only see healthy options... There are so many out there that we overlook! I remember nothing in life has meaning except the meaning we choose to give it... I cannot thank Kaelin Tuell Poulin enough for providing this program.

Jenn Murphy

Learning to love myself has always been a huge struggle of mine. I'm still fighting the battle daily, but this LadyBoss program has changed my life for the better. It wasn't until I found Kaelin Tuell Poulin that for once in my life I began to see the potential I have to offer others. Every day I work on not only my physical appearance, but more so the emotional aspect of myself. I might be single but definitely not alone in my journey.

Allicia Anne Brown

Thank you Kaelin Tuell Poulin for putting together such a life-changing program. You have helped me and so many other amazing women take the first steps in changing our lives.... I've been depressed for years because of my weight. LadyBoss is the first program that has truly motivated me and stuck with me. This program is changing the way

I see myself... and others and my outlook on life. And I am so grateful for that. I love LadyBoss, I love Kaelin, and I love each and every one of you.

Charlie Wilcox

Kaelin Tuell Poulin, I just wanted to say thank you so much for this opportunity. Thanks to you, this program has helped me get my mind and body right. It has given me the confidence I thought I'd never get back. Your program is worth every last penny... I just pray that God continues to bless you in your endeavors, in helping these women achieve their goals. You truly have made a difference in mine. Thank you so much, Kaelin Tuell IFBB Pro, you truly are my hero.

BIG FAT LIES

BIG FAT LIES

by Kaelin Tuell Poulin

BIG FAT LIES: How Everything You've Been Told About Losing Weight Is Full Of Lies And The TRUTHS That Helped Me Lose 65 Pounds Without Giving Up Pizza And Ice Cream

ISBN: 978-1-946978-01-1

First edition.

Printed in the U.S.A.

© 2017 by Kaelin Tuell Poulin

Created in partnership with Bill Blankschaen and his StoryBuilders team. (MyStoryBuilders.com)

Published by Bestseller Publishing. (Bestsellerpublishing.org)

Cover design by Sarah K. Weeks.

Dedication

To my amazing husband, Brandon, thank you for showing me my true potential.

Thank you for challenging me to be better everyday. Thank you for playing every role needed to grow LadyBoss into a successful business—for being cameraman, video editor, strategist, ads manager, copywriter, mentor, CEO, my support, and my shoulder to cry on.

I can't wait to see where God is leading us and to follow you there!

I love you!

$1 + 1 = 11$

Table of Contents

Chapter 1

Who Else Wants to Lose Weight?

Everything you've been told about weight-loss is a BIG. FAT. LIE.

I know what you're thinking. Who does this girl think she is? I get it. You've tried everything to lose weight haven't you?

- Weight Watchers.
- Nutri-System.
- Weight-loss challenges.
- All sorts of diets—under 1,000 calorie a day, no carb, no fat, high fat and low carb, shakes, South Beach, Atkins— just fill-in-the-freakin blank!

How do I know? I've been there, too, and done *all* that. And none of it worked. Yep, just a couple years ago, I weighed over 180 pounds! And I'm only 5' 2"!!

I know, I know. *Seriously* overweight. By doctors' standards, body-mass index (BMI), and every other measurement, I was considered obese. But that all changed when I lost 65 pounds in just 7 months—while still eating ice cream and pizza.

Hard to believe? Maybe I should tell you a little of my story before we get into debunking all those weight-loss lies, because you and I may have a lot more in common than you think.

I know what it's like to think you've tried everything to lose weight—and it just hasn't worked. I know what it feels like to want to give up, since nothing works anyways. I've been let down by just about every kind of diet out there. So if you've ever felt any of THAT—there's hope for you.

No matter how overweight you think you are right now, you CAN lose weight—and keep it off—using the formula I discovered on my own weight-loss journey. It's not magical. It's not a fairytale. And it's not a sales pitch some guys in a marketing department dreamed up. It's real—for YOUR real life.

And it works. I have the story—and pictures—to prove it.

What's Your Story?

So what's your story?

Since I lost 65 pounds in seven months, I've heard so many success stories from other women who've lost weight—a LOT of it. And they've kept it off.

I now have the AWESOME privilege of leading a community of women who use my proven approach to lose the weight they never thought they could lose. They thought they were stuck with it. They'd tried every diet out there, taken every powder, and bought into every new workout fad. A lot of them had given up hope. But not anymore. Now they've got awesome success stories of their own and nothing but excitement about what's next in life.

That's why I asked about *your* story. I want every woman to have a story like that. I want YOUR story to truly be one you LOVE to tell. I want YOU to be in the very best shape you can possibly be—and not just so you look good.

You deserve to enjoy life to the fullest. You've got things to do on your bucket list. Your dreams weren't meant to be buried on a back shelf somewhere—they need a healthy, vibrant YOU to dust them off and go achieve them.

Maybe you tried before, but couldn't get past tough stuff that's happened in your life. Maybe you felt like you didn't have the energy or the confidence you needed to succeed. Maybe you've made more mistakes than you can count and have slipped back into bad habits every time.

Well, I'm here to tell you that you CAN do it. And that's why I think it might encourage you to hear a little of my story. I'm not all that unusual. I'm just a small-town American girl who's had to deal with whatever life has thrown my way.

So if I can do it, you can too.

Daddy's Girl

Until we figure out how we got to where we are, it's tough to know where we want to go—and how to get there. That's why I start my story back when life seemed perfect.

I grew up in rural Indiana in a one-stop-sign town—we didn't even have a stoplight. But we had a lot of corn. Mom, Dad, my younger sister, and I lived on a 200-acre farm. My dad always joked, *"Who needs boys when I have my girls,"* because my sister and I loved to fish, hunt, ride 4-wheelers and go boating with him all the time.

Partly because of all the stuff I did with my dad, I became super competitive and loved playing sports. You name it, I did it. Basketball, softball, track, volleyball—I played all of them throughout my school years. And I was pretty good at all of them. Too good for some.

With athletic success in our small high school came all the usual criticism and petty jealousy. Even in middle school, I had always been bullied. I didn't go for the cliques. I didn't choose sides. I wanted to be friends with everybody, not just in a certain group.

I was the athletic girl who was nice to the band geeks. I talked to the kids in choir, not just the jocks. I would sit with random people at lunch to make new friends. So other students accused me of trying to get everyone to like me. I was never willing to change who I was for what anyone else thought I *should* be, and I wouldn't back down from them.

Because I was good at sports, I had really, really close friends from those teams. But when I made the transition to play travel ball, not all of those friends made the teams. Many of those so-called friends stopped inviting me to their houses. When some students didn't make the varsity team at school, their parents would actually boo me from the sidelines, even though their daughters were on the JV team. *That's just nuts.*

I had to deal with cyberbullying, practical jokes designed to humiliate me, and all the rest of it. But I never let them see me sweat. I was determined to do something meaningful with my life.

When my dad heard about all of it, he gave me the best advice: *It doesn't matter if people don't like you. That's none of your business.* I decided I wasn't going to be anything less than who I am, no matter what.

Dad gave me a lot of great advice for life. I wasn't only his first-born, baby girl; I was sort of the son he never had. I wore #3 on my softball jersey because Dad was a HUGE Dale Earnhardt racing fan.

He always made me work for everything. When I was fourteen, Dad got me a truck, even before I had a driving permit. It was a 1997 blue Chevy Silverado he'd bought from the telecommunications company where he worked. It was covered in lettering and stickers. Dad said if I wanted it, he would pay for it, but I would have to do all the work on it—including removing all those stickers.

He handed me some Goo Gone, a hair dryer, and a little paint scraper. I sat there for what felt like the entire summer that year scraping them off—every *freaking* letter! It took about three weeks.

After I finished, I drove it out into the sun and—Aargh! I could still see the outlines on the paint where the stickers had been. Nooooo!! Dad just smiled and told me to start buffing. Two weeks later, my arms felt like they would fall off, but all trace of the stickers was finally gone.

We worked on the truck together for a year and a half. Before he let me have the key, he made me take the entire transmission apart and put it back together again. He gave me some sick American racing rims, and we totally tricked it out. We put kickers in the back to make some serious noise. Even my speakers glowed neon blue. It was the coolest thing that ever hit the streets of New Washington, Indiana— our pride and joy.

Then one winter day during my sophomore year, something happened that changed everything. While dad and I worked on my truck, he suddenly collapsed in the driveway and struck his head.

From Good to Bad

My dad had been diagnosed with lung cancer a year earlier—two softball-sized masses in his chest. He'd only had a horseshoe patch of hair left at the time, so he'd shaved it off when he started chemo. He was never really the same after that treatment, even though the cancer went into remission. He used to be always on the go, working super hard in the yard, cutting grass, or fixing cars. After the chemo, he had always seemed drained and tired.

We'd sit on the couch together and watch TV—he loved the History Channel. Every year when *Band of Brothers* came on, we'd do nothing but watch for seven days. That was our thing, me and my dad.

In spite of it all, he'd made it through treatment for the lung cancer. It was in remission. He was a survivor. Or so we thought. After he collapsed in the driveway, we learned the truth: the cancer was back—brain tumors the size of golf balls. That's when it started to get real for me.

My dad was the coolest person in the world. Calm, cool and collected, but always the life of the party. He didn't want the spotlight all the time; he just always had the perfect joke at the perfect moment. Yet he became like a ghost over the next six months as all the medications took that personality away.

As a sophomore in high school, taking classes and playing sports all the time, I kept busy. Dad kept working as best he could, so none of us really knew how quickly his health was fading.

Then one day in May, 2006, not long after my 16th birthday, my dad left for work in the morning and never came home. He had chosen to take his own life. My world would never be the same.

From Bad to Worse

Have you ever had something happen that left you feeling like you just couldn't breathe anymore? Like you had a massive weight crushing your chest that just wouldn't go away? As if you hurt so much inside that it just didn't even hurt anymore? That's what I felt then—a lot of really confusing stuff. If life's ever hit you like that, you know what I mean. If you don't, consider yourself blessed.

I felt anger. I never got to say good-bye to my best friend in the entire world. Why did he leave us this way? Over time, I've come to realize that the medications he was taking meant he wasn't himself. But back then, I wanted to know how he would have done this to me.

I felt a great weight of responsibility. Dad had drilled into me the importance of being responsible. I thought that now my mom and sister would need me to step up more than ever to be the strong one, the backbone of the family to help us get through it.

I felt like I had to be the one to protect them—and I wasn't happy about it. Here I was at age sixteen with my whole life in front of me. I didn't want the responsibility of carrying my family.

I felt like life had spun totally out of control. I wasn't quite at the age where I could get much access to wild parties and alcohol. We didn't have much in the way of drug use there in rural Indiana. So I turned to the one thing I felt like I could control and could easily get—food.

I started eating more. A LOT more. Food became my drug of choice, because I could choose when and what I wanted to eat. Nobody would tell me not to eat, so I could at least be in charge of one thing in my life.

Soon my addiction to food began spiraling out of control. Soon I was eating an entire tub of cookie dough at night in my room. I'd go out in my truck and eat an entire pizza by myself. I'd stop at McDonald's twice a day. I was so unhappy with myself.

Over the next year I put on about 10 to 15 pounds. I kept playing sports—basketball, softball, volleyball, you name it. Practicing twice every day kept my weight from getting out of control. Over the course of my senior year, I gained another 10 to 15 pounds. That's almost 30 pounds in two years—even while I was playing sports most of that time. Not good.

In my junior year, our basketball team won our regional championship. In Hoosier country, that was a pretty big deal. Inside I was feeling numb to the world, but at least I had sports. But then things took a turn for the worse.

In my senior year, our team was a favorite to go all the way to the state championship. I had continued to pile on the pounds, in spite of staying active. During a practice right before the playoffs started, I stole the ball, spun, and threw the ball down the court.

Except my knee didn't turn with me. In an instant I had ripped up my entire knee—ACL , MCL, meniscus—you name it, I blew it out.

It was *game over* for me. In fact, the entire season was done. I had to come face-to-face with the reality that I would never play basketball again.

Whatever Comes after *Worse*

I don't know what stuff has happened to you in life, but we've all got struggles. Don't let anyone ever tell you otherwise. No matter what you see on Facebook, no one has a perfect life. Sometimes life hits us upside the head—again and again—until we think we can't take anymore—and then it hits us AGAIN!

It was my senior year in high school—supposedly the best time of life—and everything that had defined me to that point had been taken away. First, I lost my dad, and then I lost my ability to do the one thing that sort of kept me sane.

Execution is rule #1. None of the LadyBoss Lifestyle Hacks throughout this book will work if you don't DO THEM!

I laid in bed for the next two weeks on some serious painkillers. I lost a lot of weight, because I wasn't eating anything but pain pills and pizza Lunchables. Not the healthiest diet, let me tell you.

To make it all worse, some other girls on the team actually started the rumor that I was faking my injury. *What are you even talking about?* Basketball's my life! If they only knew....

When prom time came around in the spring, I was still wearing a cast. I had blown off my physical therapy, because I just didn't care anymore. I figured I would just be wearing a cast forever. About twenty of us (in a class of forty-four) rented a limo to go to prom together. Then some of the other girls chose that time to be stupid again. They kicked me out of the group. Nice.

Screw 'em, I thought. Who needs this? I'm outta here.

All You Can Eat—and Then Some!

After graduating from high school, I finally got off the painkillers—which meant I got my appetite back. I started binge-eating again, downing everything I could as I looked forward to getting out of town as quickly as possible. Fortunately, I had always worked hard to get good grades in school. It was a good thing, too. After my injury, college sports scholarships just weren't going to happen.

I chose to go to Hanover College, a pretty prestigious school in southern Indiana. It was far enough away from home to give me a fresh start, but still close to my family. It's a pretty selective school, but my grades got me in with an academic scholarship.

On the positive side of things, I did go out for the softball team. That encouraged me to reengage physical therapy and at least stay slightly active. But I had also lost something when I went away to college—*accountability.*

Not only did I not have any positive peer pressure, I got plenty of pressure to go the WRONG direction. Every night there was a party going on. Everyone expected us to eat whatever we wanted without questioning it. Away from home for the first time in my life, I became completely addicted to food.

Food at college was an all-you-can-eat buffet—every single day. Pizza, bread sticks, ice cream, milkshakes, desserts—you name it, they'd make it for you and you didn't have to pay for it! I would sit there with three plates of food and think, *Oh my gosh! What am I doing to myself?*

Three times a day I'd eat all I could in the cafeteria, but I didn't stop there. I'd go along on late-night beer runs and hit the drive-thru at Wendy's for a quadruple baconator, or grab a tasty cheesecake at Frisch's, or a five-pound bag of gummy bears at Wal-Mart—*all in the same night!* Then I'd top it all off with a tub of cookie dough ice cream.

There was no one to stop me, so I just ate and ate and ate. I would buy a huge piece of white chocolate and a bag of pretzels at Wal-Mart. Back in my room, I'd melt the chocolate, dip the pretzels in, and down the entire bag in one sitting. And that was *normal* for four years.

Over the next few years of late-night eating binges, I gained another 35 pounds until I tipped the scales at *more than 180 pounds!* Me, the super-athletic and fit girl. Ugh. If I hadn't been playing softball, I probably would have gained a lot more. I sort of knew it was happening, but chose to live that way, even though I hated every minute of it.

I remember thinking, *I'm too far gone now. I can't do anything about it. It's easier to just keep going and ignore it, than to do something.*

When my family went to the beach every summer, I wouldn't want to take off my bikini cover-up. I'd hide under an umbrella with a book,

Harry Potter of course, too afraid to get out of my beach chair, too upset about what I was doing, but not willing to do anything about it.

I was fat—5' 2" tall and over 180 pounds. But nobody ever said anything to me about it.

Awakened by Grandma

Have you ever noticed something? When people see us eating too much, they usually don't say anything—even though they're thinking, *Can you believe how much food she's eating? Man, has she put on the pounds!* Eating too much is a socially acceptable way to destroy ourselves.

Those who knew about my dad probably felt sorry for me. I don't know. I'm guessing they didn't want to make me mad. But the reality was that no one cared enough to call me on it. No one, that is, until I went to my Uncle Tim's house for Christmas in my senior year of college.

My grandma was always a super blunt person who would say what was on her mind and let the chips fall—*wherever.* (I see where I got it.) She also made the best cookies in the entire world!

That year she had made her special snickerdoodle cookies—the BEST! She'd pressed the top of each cookie with a fork, criss-cross style like always, then sprinkled them all with cinnamon and more sugar. I LOVED them. I kept downing her home-cooked treats, glad I didn't have to settle for store-bought cookies for once.

I reached for another, and another, and another when suddenly— SLAP! Grandma hit me. Seriously. She smacked my hand and said, "Do you really think you need to eat that cookie?"

Oh. My. Gosh. Did my little 80-year-old grandma just say that to me—right in front of everybody?

I was hurt—and angry. At first I thought I might cry. *Really Grandma? Did you have to make me feel so embarrassed with the whole family watching?* But then I thought, *How dare you say that to me? Who do you think you are?*

I talked to my mom about it on the hour-long ride home, telling her how shocked I was that grandma did that to me. My mom even called grandma afterwards to yell at her for doing it. But later that night as I thought about what she had said, I realized she said it because she cared about me.

And then it hit me: *You know what? She's right.* Now, I am not someone who easily admits to being wrong. But I knew then that grandma was right. *Look at all the weight I've gained! I didn't need another cookie.*

My thoughts screamed at me, I'm tired of it! I'm sick of it! I want to feel good about myself again. I want to have my confidence back. I want to love myself again.

Have you ever wanted what I was wanting that night? Is that something that you want right now? If so, stay tuned. Because that's when I decided, *I'm going to do it.*

As I lay in bed that night, I started Googling "weight transformations" on my phone. I saw stories of women who were moms, had careers, or even worked two jobs. I discovered stories of women who had survived abuse, health problems, and all kinds of challenges—and they still lost weight—60, 80, 100, and even 200 pounds!

Water consumption is THE KEY! Leave the cap off your water bottle to make it convenient to drink more!

Dang, I thought. *Grandma was right. I don't have to keep living this way. If I put my mind to it, I can do this. I can lose the weight.*

What about Your Story?

• What painful experiences have you had in life? How would you describe your response to those experiences—positive or negative?

_____

_____

_____

_____

• Do you eat to feel better? Do you eat when you're down, sad, or depressed about life? Be honest with yourself and jot down your thoughts about how you use food in your life.

_____

_____

_____

_____

• What parts of my story sound familiar to you so far? Where do you see connections with your own story?

_____

_____

_____

_____

• Are you ready to get real with yourself and lose weight? Yes or no? _____

Chapter 2

How I Lost 65 Pounds in 7 Months

Can I tell you a secret? It's something I haven't really told anyone. I guess I've tried to forget about it as much as possible. It's not easy for me to talk about it, but it might help you to know it. Because you may struggle with the same challenge.

I was pretty stressed out during my sophomore and junior years in college. On top of the emotional nightmare I was living in and physical injuries I was dealing with, I had to cope with all the typical college stress. Tons of papers to write, books to read, classes to juggle, and the social scene—all of it was just too much for me.

Food became my drug of choice, my escape from reality. I couldn't get enough. Literally. So when I was gorging myself on food during my sophomore and junior years, I became bulimic. I wanted to eat, but I wanted to lose weight so I forced myself to throw up. Disgusting, I know. I would eat a bunch of pizza and doughnuts or cookie dough and then throw up to keep from gaining weight.

I kept it secret from everyone. As soon as a meal was over, I would excuse myself to go to the restroom, always being careful to make sure no one else was around. I worked hard to keep up the appearance of normal. I started living a secret life, basically slipping away to puke so I could eat some more—and thinking no one noticed.

After a while, I sort of became aware that my friends thought it was odd that I would go to the bathroom after every meal. But I covered it up, concealed the truth about me, and kept eating—until Grandma got through.

If you're struggling with an eating disorder, know that you are not alone. You should also know that there is hope. You don't have to stay the way you are, hiding your problems and feeling like food is your master. You can take control of your life and lose the weight.

I Didn't Know What to Do

If you're at all like me, when you think about losing weight, you feel overwhelmed by how much you don't know. There are thousands of voices out there telling you all sorts of weight-loss lies.

When I woke up the morning after my encounter with Grandma, I didn't really know what to do next. I was determined to lose weight, but I didn't know where to start.

On the farm where I had grown up, good food meant a big ol' helping of meat and potatoes, followed by homemade desserts so rich you could feel the pounds piling on your hips. Every. Single. Night. I thought "healthy food" was a McChicken sandwich from the McDonald's drive-thru because it had chicken in it instead of beef. There was so much I didn't know.

One thing I did know—the power of habits. My years in sports had taught me that the key to doing anything well is practice, practice, practice. I knew the eating habits I had were horrible. I ate fast food two to three times every day. I drank ten Cokes a day. I lifted my textbooks from the floor to my bed and called it exercise. Clearly, I had issues.

My mind returned to the years before my dad's death, back when I was fit and athletic and felt I could do anything. If I was going to make a change, I knew I needed to change my habits.

That morning after I had made the decision to lose the weight, I woke up and made the second major decision: I chose to watch TV every day for at least 30 minutes. What?! I started losing weight by watching TV? Well, not exactly.

I figured that since I was already watching TV every day, why not work out while I watched? So I chose to create a new habit: exercise every day for at least 30 minutes while watching my favorite television shows. Walking Dead, The Office, Jeopardy—it didn't matter what show it was, I was going to be moving while watching it.

I figured I could use my time better than browsing Facebook or Instagram, and if I could sit on the couch for six hours on the weekend watching Netflix, I could workout for 30 minutes while watching something. I made the commitment with myself to be at the gym every day and work out for at least 30 minutes.

There was no one to guide me on this journey to lose weight. When I first walked into the gym, I almost turned around and walked right back out. I had no clue what to do with all the equipment I saw there. And I didn't want to look stupid. I know I should have asked questions, but I didn't want anyone to know I had no idea what I was doing. And, to tell the truth, I didn't want them to notice *why* I was there.

Working out in the morning will release endorphins and give you more natural energy for the rest of the day.

I got a little help from the guy I was dating at the time who was a personal trainer. But, honestly, I just started watching YouTube videos while I was on the elliptical. While I worked out, I watched a lot of other people workout to see how they were doing it. I studied how they used the equipment I saw around me in the gym. I watched how they worked out and learned why they did what they did. Once I became confident enough that I didn't feel like a moron, I would try using the same machines they did. And it worked.

Slowly but surely, I began to learn. Soon what had once seemed overwhelming began to feel familiar. As my fear slipped away, my confidence came back. I began to feel as if I knew what I was doing.

As my workout habit took hold, I became obsessed with something other than eating food—trying to learn as much as I possibly could about eating healthy. No joke—90% of what I learned came from searching Google non-stop to learn, learn, learn. Knowledge is power.

I'd find lists of healthy food choices and look at pictures of healthy dinners and then go to the college buffet options and recreate those dishes. I became obsessed with learning as much as I could, because I felt like I couldn't make a change if I didn't know *everything*. I know now that I was wrong.

The truth is that you can start from wherever you are and take the first steps today without becoming an expert by tomorrow. But back then, I felt like I had to learn it all. I didn't want to give myself any excuse to fall back into unhealthy habits. So I became obsessed with looking at everything: what's a complex carb? What's the difference between a healthy fat and regular fat? What's a starchy carb? I researched every diet I could find trying to figure all this stuff out.

Here I was, a girl from a Midwest farm town who never heard anything called "healthy" but steak and potatoes, researching fat burners. It was all so new to me, but I dove in and soaked up all I could.

Afraid to Ask Questions

Looking back on those first few months of my weight-loss journey, I wish I had found the courage to ask more questions and enlist the help of others who could guide me. But I was afraid to say anything.

Maybe you know what that feels like? When you walk in the gym, you're already intimidated because you don't know what you're doing, but don't want anyone else to know. Plus, you're so self-conscious about your weight that you're pretty sure everyone else is judging you for being there in the first place.

Can I tell you another secret? I've been on both sides of the gym workout spectrum now—overweight and fit—and the truth is that the fit people think they're being judged by the overweight people. And the overweight people think they're being judged by the fit people.

What I've learned is that you can't let what other people think control your life! All people need love. No matter who you are and what you look like, you are just as special as anyone else in the gym. And that's the truth. So don't worry about what the person next to you is thinking about you and ask for help. I wish I would have asked for help sooner.

I Googled "healthy recipes," "healthy breakfasts," "healthy *whatever*," and then I would try to make it happen. Because I didn't know that much, I literally stuck to the same meals every day to form new eating habits while still at college. For breakfast I had a 4-egg omelet with turkey, veggies, a little melted cheese, but no oil. For lunch I had chicken and broccoli with salsa on top of the chicken. I ate the same thing for dinner but with a salad on the side. I thought chicken and broccoli must be healthy, so I just stuck to the same things every single day. I knew it had to be better than pizza, fried cheese sticks, and cookie dough ice cream.

Then I did something important, even though I didn't realize it at the time. I went public with my weight-loss journey. I told everyone, "I'm gonna lose 20 pounds in the next three months!" I posted my goal on Facebook and Instagram. I started documenting the whole thing. Every workout, every meal, every step of the journey, I put it out there. I was completely transparent about the whole thing—I just posted the realness. And it went viral on Instagram!

It wasn't pretty, trust me. I'd post videos of me on a cardio machine, sweating my face off, feeling like I was dying with captions like, "I don't want to be here! I'm here anyway! I'm killing it—what's your excuse?"

People started sharing the pics and videos, tagging their friends who were going through similar struggles. I'd post my meals for the day, my workout, my cardio, my motivational quote for the day—I shared all of it with the world. Talk about transparency! It was scary at first, but it made all the difference.

Pretty soon, it got to the place where if I forgot to post a workout for the day, people began asking if I was ok. "Did you not go to the gym today? Did you not do cardio?" I assured them I hadn't dropped out and shared pics from that day's workout. I figured if I posted my story and all the stuff I was learning that helped me, maybe it could help someone else.

I did that every single day, day in and day out, for months. I went from having 50 followers on Instagram to eventually having over 30,000 followers. I credit it all to my total transparency about the process—my success, my failures, whatever.

What I've seen with a lot of so-called fitness experts is that they only show their wins. They show you how great they look in a new, smaller dress size, but not about the workout they did to get there. So many of them say they want to help women lose weight, but they don't share what they actually eat during the day or how many reps they do on which machines. And never once do you see them having a really bad day but still making it to the gym for a workout. You don't see any of the crap in their lives, just the flash and sparkle.

Here I was just being totally transparent and open about the whole thing because I wanted some accountability for myself. What I realized later was that so many women—women like you—just want *real*. They don't want the glitz; they want results.

So I posted everything on Instagram and soon found myself surrounded by a community of women like me who wanted to take control of their weight and live a healthier lifestyle *for real*. Even today I hear from women who've lost 20, 30, even more than 40 pounds just from what they learned on my Instagram account for free. *That's awesome!*

The Resistance *Without*

Having support from people online encouraged me to keep moving forward on my new path in my final semester of college, especially on days when I didn't feel like it.

I know some people say you should have a workout partner, but I don't think it's a good idea. It's too easy to become dependent on that person. If that person's schedule changes unexpectedly and he or she has to work late or do something with family, it gets easier for you not to go either. If someone is at the gym at the same time as me, great. But I don't want to be depending on someone else for my own healthy living lifestyle.

But I've got to tell you, what surprised me most about the journey was all the resistance I got from people who I thought were my friends. Instead of encouraging me to lose weight, work out, and eat healthier, they did just the opposite. The funny thing is that when I was gorging myself on food, puking in the bathrooms, and gaining over 60 pounds, no one said anything. But once I began making progress and started losing weight, all the critics started coming out, like they were trying to pull me back in to bad habits again.

When I was first trying to eat and live healthier, people would give me a hard time about it. "What?! Why are you eating a salad?" Even when they knew I was trying to lose weight, they would pressure me to eat junk food. "Here! Have a brownie," they would say, shoving the chunk of chocolate in front of my face. "You know you want nachos, Kaelin! Look at all the melted cheese on top—eat some with us! You're not gonna have ice ream? Are you crazy?!" The worst was when they tried to guilt me into caving in: "Oh, you think you're sooo good because you're not eating ice cream?"

What the—! I could *not* believe it! Why were all these people who were supposed to be my friends giving me such a hard time when I'm obviously trying to lose weight? Here I was trying to get my life back together and all they wanted was to shove cookies in my face!

I didn't understand it then—but I do now. You can call this another secret if you want, but here's the truth about resistance you will get from people on your weight-loss journey. When people see you changing, they look at their own lives and don't like what they see. Rather than doing the hard work of fixing themselves, they try to tear you down instead.

It's the same petty stuff that happened to most of us in middle school. People subconsciously try to tear you down to make themselves feel better. If they can get you to do what they're doing, they'll feel comfortable again. If they can see

> Don't compare your progress to anybody else! Everybody's body and results are different! Take ownership of your results and your progress.

you eating a brownie instead of a salad, or downing nachos and ice cream instead of chicken and broccoli, they'll feel better about failing. But when they see you succeeding and sticking to it, they realize they could do it too—but they choose not to.

Bottom line: your effort makes them realize it's a choice—and they're making the wrong one. I learned the hard way that people can't stand coming face-to-face with that reality. It makes them have to acknowledge that they are choosing to weigh what they weigh. They are choosing to eat cookies while you eat a salad. They are choosing an unhealthy lifestyle while you take a better path. They see it happening right in front of them, and they can't avoid the obvious—so they try to get you to go back to how you were so they'll feel better about themselves.

You can't let their fears stop you. I realized the hard way that I couldn't let my friends or family make my lifestyle choices for me. I could choose to change my life, lose weight, and live a healthier and happier life.

The choice was all mine.

The Resistance *Within*

"You are the most influential person you will talk to all day." I came across that quotation from Zig Ziglar during that season when I felt beat up by people around me.

Not only did I get criticism from the outside, I heard it every day inside my own head. I knew I had to change the negative self-thoughts I said to myself if I was going to succeed. Some of the biggest resistance I faced—more than opposition from other people—was the stuff I told myself.

I began diving into the motivational teachings of Zig Ziglar, Jim Rohn, and Tony Robbins. I soon found another key to success—positive affirmations. I began writing on my mirror the things I wanted to tell myself every single day: "I am awesome! I can lose the weight! I'm an A student!" Even after I left college I kept doing it in my apartment in Indianapolis, pouring positive thoughts into my mind every day. Every time I saw them on the mirror I would read them out loud to myself. I soon noticed a dramatic change in the way I thought about myself.

I realized that we usually ask ourselves the wrong questions. Tell me if these sound familiar: *Can I really do this? Should I eat that? Should I go for a run?* These are negative questions that make it too easy to give in and say no to the good. Instead of letting myself ask bad questions, I chose to give myself awesome answers: *I'm having a good hair day! I'm on fire today! I have a lot of energy! I'm going to have a great workout today!*

What I discovered is that when you repeat these positive statements in your life, your brain hears them as true. The more you speak them to yourself, the more they become truth in your life. You can choose what your own mind hears.

So stop asking yourself negative questions inside your own mind like, "Why am I ugly, fat, and unloveable?" When you're tempted to go there, give yourself a positive affirmation: "I'm awesome! I have energy, and I feel great! I'm beautiful! I love myself!" Trust me. Watch how your mind changes, your mood changes, your career changes, your entire life changes—all because you stop bogging yourself down with all the negative crap.

If you keep telling yourself you can't do it, a week later you'll be done. You'll fail before you even start. So many women fail to lose weight because they don't believe change is possible. They tell themselves it can't happen, then it doesn't happen. It's a self-fulfilling prophecy. But if you can do something that will result in your weighing more, then you can do something to lose the weight, too.

When I tell women on my webinars how beautiful and awesome they are, so many of them start crying because no one ever tells them that, not even themselves.

In my own weight-loss journey, I had to resist not only critics who tried to trip me up, but the lies I told myself in my own mind. But once I made the decisions and realized that success was possible, I kept taking the next step. I formed healthy living habits and shifted my lifestyle. I stopped running from the pain in my past and started running toward a better life where I could be of more help to others.

In seven short months, I lost 65 pounds—and I looked and felt great!

The Power of Habits

Over the course of those seven months, I came to understand the power of habits. Of course, as an athlete, I knew repetition was the key to getting results. But I had never fully realized how powerful eating and exercise habits could be if I harnessed them for good. Losing weight is easy to do, but it's even easier not to do.

Write your goal on your bathroom mirror with a dry erase marker so you can see it every morning.

We're all creatures of habit, whether for bad or good. Because you are the sum total of your habits, you will never change your life until you change what you do daily. Repetition equals results.

I learned I had to replace bad habits with good ones. I couldn't simply stop eating junk, I had to start eating healthy food. I had to develop new habits because habits would either be my worst enemies or my best friends. I had to replace destructive habits with healthy living habits until I no longer consciously thought about most of the healthy choices I needed to make.

The first time you do something healthy, it's like a trickle of water running down a sandy beach. It doesn't make much of a difference the first time. But over time, that little stream creates a deeper and deeper groove.

I love walking women through the process of understanding how to harness habits now as part of the LadyBoss Ultimate Transformation Academy. What I've learned from experience is that each of us must do three things to change our habits once we've identified unhealthy ones:

1. Arrest the damaging behavior by unidentifying yourself with it. Tell yourself you are NOT a binge-eater. You are not lazy. You are awesome, hard-working, and getting healthier and more fit every day. The more disconnected the old habit becomes from how you see yourself, the easier it will be to end it.

2. Replace the damaging behavior with a new behavior that better serves your goals. For example, instead of sitting on the couch watching TV, watch your favorite shows while enjoying a cardio workout.

3. Condition the new behavior to make it automatic.

- **Remind** yourself with a cue of some sort, like an alarm that goes off every three hours reminding you to eat something healthy.
- **Rehearse** your new habit in your mind first, then do it. Again and again.

- **Praise** yourself every time you do it. If repetition is the mother of all skills, then praise is the father. Rewards are like rocket fuel to the habit-forming process.

I found it helpful to write down my habits, both the negative and destructive ones and the new behaviors I wanted to replace them with. I encourage you to do the same. The more intentional you get about your healthy living journey, the more success you are going to enjoy in living out your new story!

What about Your Story?

- Let's be honest. Have you ever struggled with an eating disorder? If so, have you sought help to overcome it? Don't let embarrassment stop you from taking care of yourself. It's ok to ask for help.

- What eating and exercise habits do you have? Are they positive or negative? Take a moment to think about your daily habits and list them here. Remember, you'll never be fully motivated to change until you hate the habits that got you into trouble in the first place.

_____

_____

_____

_____

- Have other people given you a hard time when you've tried to lose weight in the past? List the words you let discourage you in the past on the lines below. Then choose not to let the fears and failures of others keep you from living a happier, healthier life.

_____

_____

_____

_____

- How do you talk to yourself about yourself? If you are the most influential person you will talk to all day, do your words ask negative questions or set you up for success with positive answers? Take a minute to write down words or phrases that would encourage you on your weight-loss journey. Write down those positive affirmations and post them where you will see them throughout the day!

_____

_____

_____

_____

- Write down your habits that you know are not healthy. Write down how you can Arrest and Replace them. How can you condition yourself to adopt the new habits? Be as specific as possible. Visualize it and then DO it!

_____

_____

_____

_____

LadyBoss Success Story

Brittany Karas, Spokane, WA

I entered college weighing 130 pounds and quickly gained 55 more. It was my second year of college when I realized that I was unhealthy and unhappy. I always made excuses as to why I couldn't hangout with friends. I always made excuses about why I didn't want to go out and do the old things I loved to do.

I tried many programs, but none of the weight was coming off, and it was frustrating me. I thought I was stuck weighing 185 for forever.

It was one of Kaelin's posts about deciding to commit to your goals for you and your why that really got me thinking. I joined LadyBoss after that. I was so discouraged and had tried so many things, so I figured why not?

LadyBoss has what a lot of programs are missing. There is constant support from a group of great ladies, an encouraging leader who tells it how it is and is present in your journey, and this program is COMPLETE. It isn't just a workout, just a diet or just support. It's all three and more. This program has not only changed my body and mindset but my whole lifestyle.

In two months I'm down 35 pounds, 10% body fat and many pant sizes. I have gone from a size 13 to a size 3-5. More importantly than sizes, I have gained my smile back and my confidence. I have gained the desire to do the old things I used to do that make me happy. I have gained the desire to go spend time with friends. I have gained the desire to eat healthy and be active. I have gained the desire to show my niece and nephew the way to live a healthy life. LadyBoss has changed my life!

Chapter 3
What's Holding You Back?

85 million women start a new diet 5 times every *single year*! Obviously, a lot of women just aren't comfortable in their own bodies. They don't like the way they look in the mirror. They don't fit in their clothes. They're embarrassed or even ashamed about it, and they don't know what to do.

Here's the thing, women naturally connect body image—what's on the outside—with self-esteem—what's on the inside. Our bodies are part of who we are, so when we feel like we're not in shape physically, it affects the rest of our lives, too.

Maybe you know what that's like? You see all these fit women in commercials, and you can't help but compare yourself to them. You see how confident they look in that 30-second clip and you know *you* don't feel *that* confident. You wouldn't look *that* good in *that* dress.

You've tried everything, and nothing seems to work. You're sick and tired of being sick and tired. You know you *need* to be healthy. You know you *should* be healthy. You believe deep down inside that you *deserve* to be healthier. But every option out there seems like it sells you a short-term solution to a long-term problem. *Quick-fix, instant burn, super shred, 6 weeks, 3 weeks, ten days*—all of it promises immediate results. Even when you make a little bit of progress, it doesn't last long, and you end up feeling like a bigger failure in every way than when you started. Ugh.

Maybe you tried that special shake diet, but quit because it just wasn't something you could continue long-term. Maybe you were one of those women who bought the latest gadget that promised to trim the weight away in 30 days *guaranteed*, but you lost both the receipt and your motivation by the end of the month. Or maybe you signed up for that expensive program with meal plans and calorie counters only to feel so overwhelmed and alone that you went right back to downing a tub of ice cream to ease your pain. Believe me, I've been there.

But it doesn't have to be this way. Losing 65 pounds in 7 months taught me that the solution wasn't to find *the one thing* that would make me lose weight fast. To lose the weight and keep it off, I realized that I needed to confront my demons and make specific and sustainable lifestyle changes.

In the chapters that follow, I'll share more of the secrets I learned— and the lies about weight-loss I exposed along the way. However, the most significant change I experienced as a result of losing all the weight wasn't what happened to me on the outside. Sure I dropped 12 pant sizes. I stopped feeling self-conscious about how tight my clothes were on me. I stopped wishing everyone would ignore me and actually wanted them *to* notice me.

Most Starbucks drinks have more sugar than FOUR candy bars. Yes you read that right. The BEST Starbucks drink alternative order is: Cold Brew with almond milk, 2 packets of stevia, and sugar-free vanilla syrup.

But it was more than that. I got my confidence back. I started walking with more purpose. I started daring to dream again. I began acting as if I could do great things. I started believing the impossible just might be possible once again.

Chasing My Impossible Dream

I don't know what your dreams are, but we've all got them. Some of us have buried our dreams pretty deep under layers of disappointments and feelings of failure. When I started experiencing weight-loss success and got my confidence back, I started rethinking my thinking. I found hope again. I dusted off those dreams and started replacing negative questions like "How could I ever do that?" with positive ones like, "What if I did *that*?"

Of course my story will be different from your story. The impossible dream I chose to pursue first probably won't be yours. Whatever your dream is, know that the impossible is more possible than you know when you get serious about following the proven formula for making healthy lifestyle changes.

Here's what happened to me once I started enjoying weight-loss success. Once I had lost all the weight, I started exploring strength training and learning more about building muscle mass. I had no plans to do anything else with it until someone made a comment to me after seeing how much weight I had lost as a result of my daily workouts.

"It's not like you're going to be a competitive bodybuilder or anything." *Whoa*, I thought. *Are you suggesting I* can't *do something? Here I am a first-born, driven-to-succeed girl who just rediscovered life again, and you're saying something isn't possible? I don't think so.*

Losing all the weight had restored my self-confidence. I started thinking about what it might be like to tackle the challenge of competing as a figure bodybuilder. Once I started thinking about it, I seemed to run into people everywhere telling me I should compete. My online friends who'd followed me on my journey kept encouraging me to compete in a figure bodybuilding competition.

If you're not familiar with the bodybuilding world—which at that point I wasn't either—figure competition isn't about getting ripped with bulging muscles. It's about muscle toning and development, body shape, stage presence and presentation. Judges are looking for the best overall physically fit and athletic physique, not the person who can lift the most weights.

Finally, I must have had a wild hair day or just too much caffeine one day, because I posted on Facebook that I was going to compete in a figure bodybuilding competition—*in the next 90 days!*

As soon as I posted it I thought, *What did you just do, Kaelin? Are you nuts?!* I hadn't even thought it through. I so wanted to delete that post right then and there. It was like I heard the old, fat Kaelin screaming in my ear that it just wasn't possible. But then the new Kaelin, the one that weighed 65 pounds less and knew she could tackle any challenge, screamed back: *You can do this! Let's take it to the next level!!*

I was in. But I only had 90 days until the competition. Here I was, a total rookie who could barely find her way around the gym less than a year earlier, needing to get ready to go onstage with women who had devoted their lives to competing. I didn't know what to do, but I had regained my confidence and knew I could find a way.

I found a body-builder friend to coach me through the training— what muscles to develop, how to pose, what to do when I got there so I didn't look like a complete idiot. I drove two hours each way to do a serious workout with him every Saturday.

I created a checklist of foods I could eat and stuck to it. Egg whites for breakfast, then a rice cake with almond butter, followed throughout the day by tuna and green beans, chicken and green beans, tuna and spinach, and then more egg whites to end the day. That's what I ate for twelve weeks. My goal was simply to get on the stage and prove to myself that I was back and ready to tackle anything.

At the end of those twelve weeks, I headed to the Kentucky Derby Classic, hosted by the National Physique Committee. I felt so lost there, wandering around backstage trying to figure out which line to stand in. There were so many women there with years of experience ahead of me who were quick to remind me that I belonged at the back of the line. I didn't care. I was so nervous that I just listened to my music and stayed covered up until it was time to walk on stage.

The place was packed, standing-room only. Thousands of people watched as I stepped out onto the stage, grinning so wide my face hurt. I remember thinking, *I did it. I made the journey from 180 pounds to a new me.* No matter what happened in the competition, I knew I had won!

Then something completely unexpected happened. After we all completed our performances, the judges called my number for first call out. Then they called it again—Best of Class for my height! I was blown away! I put my hands over my face in shock as I walked out. They handed me a sword, the usual trophy given to winners in bodybuilding. The whole place went crazy as news of my weight-loss journey had spread. I just focused on making sure I kept smiling—and breathing,

Because I won my height class, I got to come back out with the four other height class winners later. Those women just looked freaking amazing! All I could think was *I can't believe I even get the opportunity to be here.* And then they called my number again!

I literally stopped breathing and thought, *Holy crap!* I had won my class *and* best overall in my very first event, which meant I was headed to Junior Nationals to try to earn my Pro card. Unbelievable! I was blown away, because it's just unheard of for someone to win the first show—and have it be a qualifying show for Junior Nationals, no less.

My online community went nuts, congratulating me and sharing in the success, because so many of them had followed my journey. Then it hit me: Junior Nationals was only four weeks away. I actually had bodybuilding pros tell me not to go. They told me it would cost a lot of money, and I would only be on stage for ten seconds—what was the point? It's all about who's competed the longest, they told me, and that certainly wasn't me. I was just a small-town girl whose grandmother had awakened her from a self-destructive pity party.

What the heck, I thought. *Someone's got to win. Why not me?* So I put my head down for another four weeks and trained. I knew I would be going up against women who competed every weekend for years. I was determined to give it my best to prove to myself that I had left my self-destructive ways behind.

When I arrived at the event in Chicago, I was both super intimidated and super excited—at the same time. I was there to win, but just being there and knowing I did my best was a win in so many ways. I remember walking out on stage with all the girls in my height class—the best in the nation. And then they called my number—#1 in my class!

It took three days for the win to sink in. In only my second bodybuilding event—a Junior National event—I had won *first* in my class, which meant I had set a new world record by earning my IFBB pro card in record time. The previous record had been held by Erin Stern, the Arnold Schwarzenegger of the female body building world. She had done it in three events.

Earning my IFBB pro card was like being drafted into the NFL. I became one of the couple hundred IFBB Pro athletes in the world! All because Grandma had loved me enough to slap me and tell me *No*.

So What's Your Dream?

Not everyone wants to be a pro bodybuilder. You probably aren't interested in doing what I did to get on stage and compete. That's OK. Your dreams will look different. But you still have them, don't you?

Even if you've forgotten what it feels like to dream, deep down there are things you want to do in life—if only you could lose the weight, get in shape, and have the energy to do them. That's what excited me most about my record-setting win. Not only did I prove I could do it, but I proved that other women, like you, could do whatever they dreamed to be possible.

If I could make the journey from being 65 pounds overweight, depressed about the breaks in life, and addicted to food, you can lose twenty pounds, overcome whatever you're facing, and achieve your dreams, too. If you believe you can do it, map out a plan to get there, and then follow the proven formula for success, you can lose the weight and keep it off with healthy lifestyle changes.

So what's your dream? What would you want to do with your life if only you could lose 20, 30, 40, or even 50+ pounds? What challenges would you take on if you had more energy every day? What great things would you attempt if you had greater self-esteem and a healthy sense of purpose?

Maybe you would travel more, see the world, explore new places, and meet new people. Maybe you'd be more engaged with your kids and invest more time creating memories as a family. Maybe you'd go after your dream job, finally start that business, or write that book you've been talking about for years—whatever it is you want to do, today can be the day you take back control of your life!

Go ahead and give yourself permission to reconnect with those dreams! I know what it feels like to think life has passed you by, screwed you over, and abandoned you by the side of the road. I know what it feels like to turn to food for comfort—and only feel emptier after every meal.

I know what it feels like to stop feeling like that, too. You do *not* have to stay where you are right now. You can enjoy the same weight-loss success I did—and you do not have to become a bodybuilder. You can follow your own dream and achieve your goals using the same formula I used and will share with you in the next section. Imagine looking great—and knowing it! Imagine feeling great—and showing it! Imagine the very best version of you, no longer hiding behind baggy clothes and oversized excuses.

If you want to live again, stick with me. But get ready to get real. Because we're going to confront the biggest lies about weight-loss and BLOW. THEM. UP.

In the next few chapters, I'm going to reveal to you how I did it—and how you can do it too. The formula at the heart of the process isn't just for bodybuilders or gym rats. How do I know? Because thousands of ladies like you have already put it to work and achieved phenomenal results.

Carry a protein bar (my favorite brand is Quest) at all times in your purse. Eat it when you're hungry instead of stopping at the gas station.

What's Holding You Back?

- Let's talk about YOUR dreams. Do you have a bucket list of things you want to do, see, or accomplish in life? If not, why not? Take a few minutes to reconnect with your dreams and use the lines below to capture them on paper.

- Try this activity. From your dream list above, choose the one dream that really excites you most. On the lines below, describe what it will be like when you achieve that dream— who will be there, how will you celebrate, and how will it make you feel? Be as detailed as possible as you imagine what it will be like when you achieve your dream!

- **Step 1:** As you envisioned yourself achieving that dream, what excuses popped into your head? Did you think of reasons you could never achieve your dream(s)? Let's name those excuses right now and list them here in Step 1, because as we move forward, you're going to leave them here with your extra weight!

Excuses	Answers
_____	_____
_____	_____
_____	_____
_____	_____
_____	_____

- **Step 2:** Remember to give yourself positive answers! For each of the excuses you listed above, cross it out and write a positive answer next to it. For example, if you wrote "I don't have enough time to work out," cross that out and write, "I have all the time I need to get and stay healthy!" Use these as part of your daily positive affirmations to start taking control of your weight-loss journey.

LadyBoss Success Story

Alexandria Blue, Garden Grove, CA

I've been on this journey for 4 months. I have a toddler son, and I'm married to such an awesome, supportive husband. I'm 27 years old, so my high school reunion is right around the corner. I had previously decided I wouldn't go because I wasn't happy with how I looked. What a cop-out, huh? Instead of doing something about it, I just said I wouldn't go.

Well, now I can say I'm thrilled I'll be going, and can't wait to tell everyone about LadyBoss when they ask me about myself.

This month, I made myself do some deep thinking about why I am where I am, and why I have struggled with my weight the last few years. That's when I realized that, although I've only been overweight about 4 years, I've struggled with food and body image my whole life. I became obsessed with my weight in high school during my freshman year. I got heavily involved in soccer, so I was training and doing lots of cardio 5 days a week.

I saw incredible results from that, but it still wasn't enough for my unhealthy mind. I started not eating. My whole day could consist of a small snack bag of chips and a soda. And then I would beat myself up so badly for that and run extra miles to punish myself.

The scariest part is how many compliments I got daily about how great I looked, even when it got to an unhealthy look. It made it so much harder to stop! This went on for about a year. Finally, and I thank God that this happened, my little brother saw me after waking up one morning, and since I was wearing a short shirt and shorts, he saw my rib area and stomach. He was so scared for me.

He asked me, to please stop doing this. I'm scared you will die. Eat something please.

Seeing him like that made something click for me. A light bulb went off. That's the day I decided to change my life. I began eating again. Eventually, after dating my now husband for so long and getting comfortable, I started putting weight on because I went the complete opposite way with food.

Food is something that I've always had an unhealthy relationship with. It's something I've viewed as the enemy for so long. Finding the LadyBoss program has helped put food in a different light for me. I don't look at it as the enemy anymore; instead I see it as fuel needed to make my body strong and to fuel my workouts. Honestly, it's a still a struggle some days to make the healthy choice. But this is a lifestyle change, so I have forever to keep practicing.

I joined LadyBoss to become strong, to feel better mentally and physically. It wasn't about just a number on the scale getting smaller. I am also down 3 pant sizes. I started at a very tight size 16. I refused to buy 18s though. I'm now a size 10. This program has been life-changing for me as far as attitude daily, mental toughness, and a healthy mindset. I don't spend all day everyday beating myself up anymore. It's hard work, but I deserve to be healthy. I deserve to be a priority to myself. Although people can see and comment on the weight I've lost, I think the biggest thing I've taken away from this program is mental.

I'm so much happier with who I am now. I have Kaelin and the wonderful support network to thank for that. I feel like a new woman, a stronger, happier, more positive, adventurous one. I'm never going back.

Chapter 4

Be Your Own Boss

What's your weight-loss secret?

People always ask me to reveal the secrets of how I lost all the weight and transformed my lifestyle. What's the secret exercise, the secret diet, or the secret supplement? Women chase me down all the time and try to get this secret out of me, but I'm going to tell you right now what it is: the secret is *Hard. Freaking. Work.*

Nobody wants to hear the truth. They want to hear that the secret is a quick and easy fix. They want to hear that they don't have to step out of their comfort zones. They want to hear that it's going to be simple—just take one pill, eat one magical fruit from deep in the rain forest, or do this one amazing cardio routine and—poof—all your weight will disappear.

But it doesn't work that way. I know the truth doesn't make for a glitzy marketing campaign, but until you realize the truth about the lies you've been told, you'll never be free to achieve your dreams. The difference between achieving your weight-loss dream and settling for excuses is the hard work in between.

You can choose to close this book right now and brush aside what I'm telling you, but I'm telling you the truth because I care about women like you achieving success not only in weight loss, but also in life. I want your dreams to become reality, but the weight-loss industry just wants to make money off you. And if you lose all the weight, they won't make any more money. Makes sense, right?

That's why the weight-loss industry needs the next big fad—to make money off your frustration, of course. They're always telling you to stay away from some specific food or to load up on one specific vitamin. They're always trying to sell you on some new "breakthrough idea" they've "discovered" that's the new holy grail of weight-loss.

There have been so many LIES told about how to lose weight that its hard to even distinguish the TRUTH anymore, like the "No Carb Diet", the "High Fat Diet", the "Eat under 1000 calories a day diet", and all the other—pardon my French—B.S out there.

My goal in writing this book is to help rewire the thoughts you have about weight-loss and health so you can get real results right now and for years to come. I want you to enjoy a healthy lifestyle, not follow a fad designed to take your money and leave the pounds alone.

As I mentioned earlier, when I first started trying to figure out how to lose weight, I got caught up in all of this mumbo jumbo, chasing the next big "secret" to losing weight. Every time I heard the new, bigger, better way to lose the weight, I whipped out my credit card. We want to lose the weight so badly that we're willing to do ANYTHING. When we fall for the B.S., we often end up doing extremely unhealthy stuff to our bodies, ending up sick, tired, or even worse off than we already were.

Trust me, I get it. When I was 65 pounds overweight, I remember feeling so overwhelmed because I didn't know what to believe. I didn't know what was legit or what was bogus. So don't feel bad if you're like me and have tried every weight-loss "fad" out there, searching for the one thing that will actually get you results. The truth is this: there is no shortcut, no magic supplement, no "lose weight overnight" solution—no matter what celebrity tells you otherwise. Developing a healthy lifestyle is hard freaking work, but it is the only path proven to get the results you want.

Before I expose and debunk the weight-loss industry lies, I want to help you rewire your thinking about weight loss and healthy living. If you don't rewire your thinking about weight loss, then you'll continue to move in the wrong direction. You'll continue to think the wrong things about how to get results. You'll continue to do more harm than good to your body.

I want more for you. I want you to experience REAL, LONG-LASTING results. That's why I started the LadyBoss community, because I know you are capable of more. LadyBoss isn't about me—it's become far bigger, with tens of thousands of women making the decision to make a change—and enjoying weight-loss success because of that decision.

Time to Take Control

Are you a LadyBoss? Not everyone is, but everyone can be. Some women are content to let life happen to them. They give in to the pain or the fear of feeling uncomfortable and just quit—but not a LadyBoss.

Quitting is normal. A LadyBoss is *not* normal. A LadyBoss is the courageous woman inside who takes responsibility for where she's at in life. She isn't a victim of circumstances. She doesn't blame someone or something else for her reality. She doesn't make excuses or complain about what she can't change. She spends more energy doing something about it instead of telling everybody why she "can't." She chooses to respond to challenges, not just react to adversity.

A LadyBoss can have everything that matters in life and do it all without compromising who she is or her integrity. A LadyBoss realizes she shines most when she is authentic and true to herself. A LadyBoss doesn't just talk, she gets things done. She recognizes that if she wants results and success, she has to put in the work.

A LadyBoss doesn't aim to please others' expectations. She aims to be the best version of herself she can be. A LadyBoss doesn't listen to all the negative critics and haters around her who are afraid she will succeed and expose their feeble excuses. A LadyBoss focuses on what she wants instead of on why some people think she won't succeed.

A LadyBoss is a no B.S., take action, get it done, no compromise woman who values her integrity, confidence, self-worth, and doesn't change who she is for anybody. A LadyBoss is in control of her situation, her health, her body, her life, and, in turn, her destiny.

Becoming a LadyBoss is a new reality you choose to step into, your confident alter ego. It means putting aside all your doubts, all your fears, all your excuses, and every reason you think you can't do it.

When you choose to be a LadyBoss, you choose to take charge of your life. You choose to regain control of your own destiny. Because you *can* do it. You can lose the weight. You can enjoy a happier, healthier lifestyle.

But you *must* choose. The decision to change is all yours. You have to decide to lose the weight. You have to decide to make the lifestyle changes. No one else can do it for you.

Set an alarm to stand up at work every 30 min. The more you stand, the more calories you burn. Don't be sedentary!

Choosing to Change

When I laid in bed that night after Grandma got my attention, I made the choice. I didn't have all the answers. You don't need to have them all either. I didn't fully understand my *why*. I'll explain why that matters in the next chapter, but you don't have to be clear on your *why* either to make the decision to change. I didn't even know all the reasons why I had let myself slide. You may not totally understand how you got to where you are now.

Don't let any of that stop you from making the decision *right now* that you will not stay where you are! Decide not to settle for the status quo anymore! You're better than that! It's time to choose a different path forward.

Choosing to change is a powerful move. Once you choose to discover the new you, your perspective on challenges begins to change. For example, one of the biggest complaints I hear from women is about stress: *I'm stressed about work. I'm stressed about time. I'm stressed about my kids. I'm stressed about making it to the gym.* Just fill in the blank with your own stress excuse.

The more you tell yourself you're stressing out all the time, the more you're going to stress out. Once you make the decision to change, you don't sweat the small stuff. And let's face it, it's almost *all* small stuff. When you start stressing out, your cortisol levels go up. Your body hangs on to fat, because it thinks it may need it to survive. Your own body subconsciously self-sabotages your efforts when you haven't made a clear decision to change.

Once you choose to change, you recognize an unhealthy response to stress because it doesn't fit with your new lifestyle. You can then look for healthy ways to defuse that stress. For example, a great way to minimize stress that I learned from Tony Robbins is to replace that stressful reaction with a grateful response. Whenever you start to feel stressed out or anxious, stop and think about three things you're grateful for today. They don't have to be huge things. They can be as small as a raindrop or as big as your relationship with your spouse. Thinking about those things brings you back to a mentally and emotionally awesome place. The good feeling of gratitude lowers your stress levels and positions you to succeed. I kick-start my day with this simple practice every morning as a preventative move and end each night the same way with my husband to cure any thought-toxins I soaked up throughout the day.

You are the only one who can decide you want to take this weight-loss journey. You're the only person in control of your actions. I can't do it for you. Your friends can't do it for you. Your personal trainer can't do it for you. You are the only one who can decide, because you are the only one who can put in the work. You are the only one that controls what goes into your body. You're the only one that gets to talk to yourself inside your head all day mentally. You're the only one in charge of you.

If you are going to become a LadyBoss and succeed, you've got to take control and know you are the one responsible for the decisions. You are the only person that can go get it done. You can't make a weight-loss wish, blow out your birthday candles, and then expect the UPS driver to knock and say, "Hey, here's your package for the 30 pounds you wanted to lose this year." That's not the way this works.

You know my story already. I tried anything and everything to lose the weight I had gained before making the REAL decision to change. When I weighed 180 pounds, I told myself it wasn't my responsibility. I told myself it was out of my control. There was nothing I could do about it. I'm too tired to go to the gym. I have a slow metabolism. I'm big-boned. It runs in my family.

I had every excuse in the world as to why I couldn't lose the weight. I blamed everything outside of me instead of taking responsibility for myself. The day everything changed for me was that day I took responsibility for all the junk I was putting in my mouth, and the exercise that I wasn't doing.

In the earlier chapters, I shared some of the painful stuff that sent my life spinning off-course. I encouraged you to write down the reasons you let your own weight get out of control. I asked you to do that because I know first-hand the power of taking responsibility for your own current situation. As long as your physical health is someone else's fault, there's nothing you can do about it is there? You'll just keep blaming it on someone, something, or anything rather than choosing to make a change. Until you realize that you've never *accidentally* eaten anything, you'll keep offering excuse after excuse as to why you weigh too much.

If you're not taking responsibility for your decisions, you will never succeed. You can either have the excuses or you can have the results. Once you quit playing the blame game and choose to change, you'll realize you can change your actions. And when you change your actions consistently, you'll change your results.

Keep your metabolism working for you by setting several alarms on your phone throughout the day as reminders to eat a healthy snack such as: Handful of almonds, an apple, carrots w/ hummus, protein bar, 2 rice cakes, or a 2-Go tuna packet.

What's Holding You Back?

- Are you ready to make a change? Are you willing to choose a healthier path in life? Are you truly disgusted with the habits you've allowed to self-sabotage your dreams? You must choose to make a change. If you're serious about losing weight, make your decision now and record it on the lines below. Then sign your name to seal your choice to embrace the new you!

  I choose _____

  Your Signature_____ Date _____

- Start a healthy habit. If you struggle with stress, start and end your day with gratitude instead. When you wake up, think of three things you're grateful for. End the day the same way. Set an alarm if you need to in order to get used to the habit. Do this for just a week and I promise you'll notice a huge difference in your stress levels throughout the day.

Reminder: Don't forget to review your positive affirmations. Add the three grateful things practice to your positive affirmations to start and end your day in a positive way.

LadyBoss Success Story

Jessie Tootle, Tallahassee, FL

2016 was a big year in my life, so I had a lot to reflect on for my April birthday. My husband graduated college, was commissioned with the Air Force, and became an officer. We moved into a new city and state. Everything changed!

I started to think about what I wanted to go back to school for and what I wanted my life to look like. I decided I wanted to look into joining law enforcement, to serve my community and set a strong example for any future kids we have. I knew I wasn't in the physical shape I needed to be in, but I made an excuse and put it off for another day.

That same night, I weighed myself and discovered I was the heaviest I'd ever been (210!). I was beyond heartbroken. I cried and buried my emotions in ice cream. How was it possible I gained so much weight? I woke up the next morning to see a post from a friend who used Kaelin's program with amazing results. She's now a manager at a gym and competes in obstacle course races in her free time, a total BA! She was so in love with herself and proud of her accomplishments that she filled me with motivation. I decided I never wanted to feel so much self-hate ever again; I wanted to feel the way she did about her body! I was going to do whatever it took to take care of myself.

I enrolled in May, and started to make subtle changes. I used to sleep 12 hours a day. I would eat candy and garbage "food" everyday, and don't even get me started on how much Coke I was consuming. I would skip breakfast, just have a 44-ounce Coke instead, eat awful food for lunch, with another Coke, stop by a gas station on my way home for a king-sized candy bar and, you guessed it, another Coke. Dinner was a joke, and I usually ate another dessert late in the night. Of course, I had no energy, and I was constantly sick.

Today, I work out every day, eat 5 times a day to fuel my body with nutrition and wholesome energy, drink a gallon of water a day, and I sleep better in 7 hours than I ever did in 12 hours before. I'm HAPPY, and I've fallen so in love with myself! I feel empowered to motivate other women and help them with the same struggles I have. I'm down 2 sizes, and I no longer fit into any of my plus-size clothing! I had to take another notch out of my watch this week; who even knew "wrist fat" was a thing?

I'm literally writing this from the treadmill, at midnight, on a Tuesday, LadyBoss style, Cardiokilla #1 (Because champions get it done)! If you would have told me 3 months ago that this would be me, I'd probably laugh in your face, because I wouldn't have been caught dead anywhere near the gym, let alone this late at night.

I'm not perfect, and I'm far from finished. I haven't had a perfect track record. But I'll never go back, everyday is a victory! Now I'm confident that I can be a great law enforcement officer!

All I can think to do is say THANK YOU, KAELIN. She has seriously CHANGED MY LIFE, FOREVER. I truly believe that Kaelin was put into my path for a reason. I can never repay her for her help, but I will tell everyone I meet about her and how much she means to me. If I could have lunch with anyone in the world, it would be her. And we would just talk, and maybe do some squats together!

Chapter 5

Find Your Why—
To Make You Cry

Why do you want to lose weight? Most women never really stop to think about what's motivating them to shed the pounds. They know they *should,* but they don't know their *why.* And that's why they fail.

A lot of weight-loss programs miss this most essential step for weight-loss. They promise phenomenal results if you'll just eat certain meals or buy their special system. But you can't start with *how* to lose weight. The truth is, you won't eat *how* you should *consistently,* if you don't know *why* you want to lose the weight in the first place. Weight-loss success starts with finding your *why.*

Other programs tell you it's all about a unique approach to your workout and exercise routine, but you won't head to the gym when there's snow on the ground or when you've had a bad day unless you're *really* motivated to do it. You can conquer any *how* as long as you have a deep burning *why.* But without the *why, how* will always fall short.

There is no shortage of negative *how* questions: *How* are you going to make time? *How* are you going to afford better food? *How* are you going to figure out a good workout plan? *How* are you going to survive the workout? *How* can you take what you're doing to the next level?

How can you lose a hundred pounds? Any of these *how* questions can take you down, but they don't have to.

You truly can conquer any *how* as long as your *why* is big enough. The journey to lose the weight and finally become the happy, healthy woman you've always wanted to be on the outside, begins with taking a look deep inside.

So why *do* you want to lose the weight? What's really driving you to do it? If you're like some women I work with, you want to enjoy your kids for as long as you can. Maybe a disease runs in your family, but you want to do all you can to make sure it doesn't become part of your story. Maybe you want to be able to be as active as possible for as long as possible to make memories with family. Whatever it is that drives you most, you have to get crystal clear about it—then harness it to help you conquer all the *how* questions that will come your way. You've got to tap into the emotions beneath it and the passion behind it if you're ever going to lose the weight. You can do this! No doubt about it. But first, you have to figure out what motivates you.

What Motivates *You?*

No one knows what motivates you, but you. Once you've made the decision to take control of your health and be your own boss, it's time to ask yourself the next question: *why* do you want to change? If you know your *why* and write it down and keep it in front of you, you'll be motivated to do what needs to be done to lose the weight—and keep it off. Any approach to weight-loss that doesn't start with your *why* is missing the point and probably setting you up for failure.

Why do you really want to lose weight and get healthy? What deep motivation pushes you to make a change? Your *why* can't be that you just want to fit back into your jeans from high school. That's not a *why*; it's just a wish. It can't be something shallow on the surface of your life.

Your *why* should literally bring you to tears as you think about it and write it down.

Your *why* should make you cry.

Is your motivation health-related? Do you want to lose weight so you don't become yet another member of your family who dies from an obesity-related illness? Is there someone in your family suffering from that right now? Do you *not* want to be that person? Or are *you* the one suffering because you haven't been able to get your weight under control?

Maybe your motivation is more about self-esteem. Do you want to love your body again? Do you want to feel comfortable again with your friends at the beach? Do you want your husband or boyfriend not to be able to take his eyes off you?

Maybe you care about helping other people. Is there pain in your past that makes you want to help other women find healing and hope? Do you want to be the person inspiring a ton of other people with your transformation journey? Do you want to lose the weight to show other people that they can do it to?

That was and is a big part of my motivation for my losing all the weight and it is front and center today. Every single day I go to the gym and do cardio, I know I have people watching. I want to inspire every single person out there to know that if I can lose sixty-five pounds, they can do it too. That's what drives me. When I think of all the woman out there who are struggling to feel better about themselves, my *why* makes me cry.

Pay yourself $1 every time you exercise. Once a month splurge on a new piece of workout clothes with the money you earned!

Your *why* has to be greater than "I want to look good in a bikini," because that's not going to get your butt out of bed on a cold morning. Your *why* should be way deeper than a surface reason for getting the pounds off. It should be deep and powerful, so it will MOVE you to take action.

If you want to succeed, you have to find your own *why* to make you cry. Whatever it is, it should literally move you to tears. It should be bigger than just yourself because most of the time we won't do it only for us, but we'll do it for our family, we'll do it to be a role model to someone else, and we'll do it to stick around and show our family how life is supposed to be lived.

Who do you want to inspire? Who do you want to be around longer for? Why do you want to lose weight—deep down inside? Once you discover your true *why*—and grab hold of it with both hands—you'll find the motivation every single day to eat and exercise the way you know you should without making excuses.

Turning Pain into Progress

As you think about finding your *why*, you might be tempted to think, *Nobody understands the pain I've gone through. People just don't get it. My situation isn't like anyone else's. If Kaelin only knew the crap I've had to deal with in life!*

I get it. Maybe you've lost someone you cared about, went through a tough divorce, or have had to endure challenges with your kids. All of us have faced different situations, but one thing I know for sure: *all of us have been through pain*. Every one of us has obstacles to overcome. Everyone has to decide what to do with those obstacles. We can react to them—and shovel in more food—or we can choose to respond in a way that harnesses the pain to do some good. We can choose to *react* or *respond*.

Stephen Covey describes a space between *stimulus*—what happens to you—and *response*—what you do with what happens to you. In that space, you and I have all the power in the world, whether we realize it or not.

So I've got to ask, how are you dealing with the pain that's come your way in life? I told you some of my story, so you would know I have some experience dealing with pain. I know what it's like to react in self-destructive ways. I started self-sabotaging, letting the pain destroy me, instead of harnessing it and turning it into something positive. Once I started waking up to what I had allowed myself to become, I realized that weighing 180 pounds was not something that would have made my dad proud.

I chose to turn that pain into something positive. I decided I didn't want to become someone who let pain serve as an excuse to roll over and die. I also didn't want to be like the sad puppy dog that everyone feels sorry for. I didn't want to live in an endless pity party. I wanted to take those things and harness them, make progress, and become someone I knew my dad would be proud of. I have no doubt in my mind that he is looking down now and happy that I haven't let the pain of losing him destroy me.

Are you letting your pain lead to bad habits or addictions like I did? Are you dealing with it or ignoring it and hoping it will all feel better if you take just one more bite? Everyone has some sort of pain, a story of devastation that tests them to either quit or find the motivation to succeed.

My commitment got tested in a big way not long after I won the bodybuilding title. I had started a sales company in the nutrition industry with my boyfriend who had recently become my fiancé. We built our business together and ended up dong extremely well, especially for two kids just out of college. We built a team that generated more than $200,000 a month in revenue. I had won the fitness bodybuilding tournament and got my pro card in record time. I was getting married to my friend and business partner. I thought life couldn't get much better at that point. Then something unexpected happened to test my motivation.

After I had achieved everything I had hoped for in weight-loss and gotten into the best shape of my life, my fiancé cheated on me. *Unbelievable, right?* When I found out, however, I didn't blame myself or fall back into thinking I was a victim. I didn't beg him to stay to work it out. Because of my success, I had acquired the confidence I needed to move on. Just like that, we were done.

But that doesn't mean it wasn't challenging. Our business had been built around his personal info, so all of it went away overnight when I broke it off. I went from insanely successful—with a monthly income of over $20,000—to totally *broke* in a single moment. I had only $200 to my name.

To make it worse, there was a national convention for our company that I had to attend as a leader. About a hundred people from our team were still looking to me for help. I had already broken up with him—and he brought the other girl to the event in front of our team. So there wasn't any way to avoid this challenge. I had to face it head-on. As a leader, I just had to shut up and suck it up. Somehow I made it through the event without punching anyone in the face—though God knows I was tempted to at times. I ended up winning an award at the event for best body transformation

> If you're eating healthy all week, have a cheat meal! 1 entree and 1 dessert of anything that you want. It will keep you sane and help reset your metabolism.

in the entire company. It was another cool moment on my journey, but afterwards, I faced another significant test.

We had just got a house together, so I couldn't stay there. I ended up just packing up my car, giving him his ring back, and finding an apartment where I could crash while I put the pieces back together again. I literally had nothing but a skillet and an air mattress. All I could afford to eat was egg whites. That was it. Nobody even knew where I was staying, so I was alone—a dangerous place, for sure.

I was back where I had started in some ways, and yet everything was different. My mentality had shifted. I had grown and developed as a person. I had learned more about me and how strong I truly was. As I sat in that apartment all alone cooking egg whites on my skillet, all the lessons my dad had taught me came back to me. I knew it would all come down to me, focusing on my *why* and choosing to respond instead of react. Either I was going to sit on my air mattress and eat ice cream to drown my sorrows or start over and rebuild. I could whine about how I only had $200, or I could dig deep to reconnect with my *why* and keep moving forward.

The thought of quitting disgusted me as I thought, *Screw this! If I did it once, I can do it again.* I had experienced so many wins, big and small. I had celebrated so much along the way—losing the weight, winning the competitions, building the business—I knew I could do *anything*.

I was so on fire that I didn't let myself wallow in self-pity, not that I wasn't tempted. I had to fight it at times, especially when I'd go to the grocery store to buy egg whites, peppers, and mushrooms to make my own frittatas. There were times I wanted to put all the healthy food back, stroll down the candy aisle, and start filling my cart with junk food. I remember really craving Cheeto Puffs and thinking no one would ever know if I gave in and went back to my old habits.

Then I slapped myself back to reality. I didn't need Grandma to get my attention by then. It had gotten easier to discipline myself to make the healthy lifestyle choices. I settled for some Quest bars as a healthy alternative, even though I really felt like buying a big bag of M&Ms and having a good cry. But I just couldn't allow myself to go back to that self-destructive place. I wasn't going to let those thoughts continue to grow in my head. I had taken the time to figure out *how* I had gone in the wrong direction before. I knew the habits to avoid and behaviors that could trigger a relapse. I knew being on my own posed a unique risk, so I had to keep my guard up. Thinking no one would ever know was one of those thoughts I had used as an excuse before.

I hated the place I had been and refused to go back. Because I had gotten in touch with my *why*—at a deep, emotional level—I know going backwards wasn't going to get me where I was determined to go. The same is true for you. Whatever may have happened to you in the past, you can ensure you keep moving forward by getting clear on what motivates you to succeed.

The Most Important Person in Your Life

So what about you? Are you turning a painful past into something positive? Are you progressing *from* it or do you keep returning *to* it? If you love your family or kids, are you doing something healthy with your life that will make them proud, or are you self-sabotaging because of circumstances beyond your control?

Can I just be totally honest and say something about the pain you feel from your past? You have to learn to let it go. You have to turn that pain into something that becomes a burning fire inside of you and use it to do something that makes your life great and helps other people around you.

You cannot change the past, but you can control what happens today and tomorrow. You've got to let go of what brought you to this point. You can't let it continue to be an emotional monkey on your back, holding you down and keeping you from success. Stop beating yourself up about what's already been done and focus on what you have to do to get to where you want to go.

Can I say something else for all you ladies who live to help other people? You have such a huge heart for other people that you're always taking care of everyone else. You're always on the go, doing things for other people. You're the supermom, the academic leader, or the go-to person in the office. Let me tell you the truth: you're not going to last long only focusing on other people. If you're giving up your health to help others in the short-term, you won't be able to help them for very long. And the help you do give won't be your best.

When you are everyone else's #1 cheerleader, but put yourself on the backburner, you're not going serve others for very long. *You* are the most important person in your life. You have to take care of *you* before you take care of anyone else. You must decide that your *why* is important enough to protect at all costs or you soon won't be able to help anyone else feel important.

And for all of you who feel like you don't qualify anymore because you've tried and failed to lose weight, know this: you *are* going to fail. You're going to mess up. You're going to get off track. Success is all about how fast can you recognize your mistake and get back on track. It isn't about perfection. You're never going to have a journey that's perfect. We all mess up, and we all fail. It's okay. As long as you're learning from it, and moving forward, that's what matters.

I'm not writing these words so you'll feel better about where you are right now. I want more for you, and you should too. *Better* begins with finding your *why*. I can show you the proven formula that works. I can debunk the lies to remove obstacles along the way, but only you can find your *why*. The new you can become a reality—sooner than you think!

The first step is yours—dive deep to discover *the why to make you cry*. Only then will you be ready to lose weight so you can start to celebrate the awesome story of *you*.

What's Holding You Back?

- Why do you want to lose weight? It's time to get clear on the *why* to make you cry. Get away from distractions, even if it's for 10-15 minutes and really think about *why* you want to lose the weight. What's your motivation? If it doesn't move you to tears, it's probably not a big enough *why*. Use the lines below or get more paper and sketch out your thoughts first. You may end up writing two to three pages about it. Distill your *why* down into a single paragraph here so you can easily find it.

  I want to reach my goal because_____

  _____

  _____

  _____

  _____

- Once you figure out your *why*, do what you have to do to keep it in front of you each and every day. If it's people you care about, set their pictures as wallpaper on your phone or put pictures on your desk and in your car. Write your *why* in frickin' lipstick on your bathroom mirror if you have to so you see it every morning. Use your imagination, but make sure you can't avoid it!

LadyBoss Success Story

Tressa Sandfort, Williamsburg, MO

When I was 4 years old, my mom noticed that I had started to get weak. I couldn't climb stairs or get up off the floor without pulling myself up with the assistance of the couch. I went to doctor after doctor and specialist after specialist.

Finally after a year or so and a couple of surgeries, I was diagnosed with an autoimmune disease called Juvenile Dermatomyositis, which is an inflammatory disease of the muscle, skin and blood vessels that affects about three in 1 million children each year.

So after years of medication, skin grafts, and people telling me that I could never keep up with the other kids physically, I believed them. I never pushed myself; I just learned to live with it. When I was 23, I was told by my dermatologist that adults who continue to carry DM into adulthood could be wheelchair bound by their early 40s. I battled depression for what could happen, but now I have had enough. My WHYS are to overcome my weight issue so I can build muscles and do the things everyone told me I couldn't do! So that I can beat the odds of being wheelchair bound, and so I can be here for my kids and grandkids without restrictions, LadyBoss style!

Chapter 6

The LadyBoss Formula

"I *love* bread!"

You've probably seen the Weight Watchers ad with Oprah Winfrey gushing about how much she *loves* to eat bread. Weight Watchers lets Oprah have it all and you can have it all, too—*if only you buy their program.*

You've got to know a lot of the money women pay for that program goes to pay Oprah for telling them how much she *loves* bread. The worst part is this: *Weight Watchers is crap.* But most women see Oprah and think it must be legit. They think they can push the easy button—join the program, eat whatever they want as long as the points add up, and they'll lose weight.

It's all B.S.

The Weight Watchers system is based on points, but an Oreo cookie is still a freaking Oreo cookie, whether it's worth two points or ten points. You could keep your points down with Weight Watchers and still eat Oreo cookies—or all kinds of bread—all day long. But eating Oreos, Pop-Tarts, and Cinnamon Toast Crunch all day won't get you a healthy lifestyle. You won't lose weight and keep it off so you can achieve your dreams.

A lot of these programs give the appearance of success, because if you restrict yourself to a certain amount of minimal calories per day, you will *lose* weight in the short-term. But then it will all come back on five-fold. These low-carb, low-calorie diets *can* give you some initial weight-loss, but twelve weeks later you've put on another ten pounds. Then you feel too embarrassed or discouraged to complain about it. They make you think it's all your fault for not sticking to the program, a program that was impossible to stick to in the first place and unhealthy on top of it all. No wonder so many women fail to lose weight and make real healthy lifestyle changes. These programs aren't intended to help them live a healthier life.

Not only do these programs make it super difficult for you to be consistent, they don't give your body the nutrition it needs to be healthy. They sacrifice long-term health for short-term success. When your body doesn't get the nutrition it needs, it goes into survival mode. Programs like the Atkins diet deprive you of carbs—what your brain needs to function. Eventually your brain will start shutting down, making it hard to have energy for your day, hold conversations, or even remember your own phone number. Once you realize its impossible for you to continue living this way and you go back to eating carbs, your body stores them as fat because it doesn't know when it will next get what it needs. To make it worse, most people go for unhealthy carbs, making the weight pile on even faster. You can easily end up putting on triple the weight you lost at first, because your body is in total starvation mode.

I tried this approach once. After I quit eating carbs for about twelve weeks, my body started

Use a heart rate monitor at the gym to measure how hard you're actually working. Apple Watch, Fit Bit, Polar, and Scosche are good options.

shutting itself down. Without complex carbs, I was running on empty. Then when I started putting complex carbs back into my diet, I gained 40 pounds in 6 weeks! Everyone thought I was pregnant because I gained weight so fast.

So here's the truth, no matter what Oprah says: you can't just focus on losing weight. You need a healthy lifestyle. Anything else is total B.S. After all, what's the point of losing weight if you become less healthy in the process?

Losing 65 pounds was really just part of my journey to a healthier lifestyle. If I had managed to lose some pounds for a while, but continued with unhealthy living habits, I could never have kept it off or gotten into the best shape of my entire life.

Living a healthy lifestyle is not about your weight. (I can almost hear your sigh of relief!) Weight affects your health, for sure, but it's not the ultimate measurement of how healthy you are. In fact, one of the biggest lies the weight-loss industry sells you is that your scale matters. It doesn't. You should throw it out. *Seriously*.

I'll explain more when I debunk all the BIG, FAT LIES you've been told about weight-loss in later chapters. For now, know that the proven formula that tens of thousands of LadyBoss women and I use is all about creating a healthy lifestyle. Most women will lose weight on the way to achieving that goal. But weight-loss itself should not be the #1 goal. It's an *awesome* by-product of following the LadyBoss Formula to a happier, healthier lifestyle.

Your Success Formula

As a result of my own intensive journey to take back control of my health, I figured out the LadyBoss Formula for healthy living success. It took a lot of trial and error, a ton of study, and, frankly, a lot of input from others on the same journey before I finally put the pieces together.

The Formula is simple, but powerful, comprehensive, yet doable. And anyone can understand it. Here it is.

(Fitness + Nutrition) x Accountability = Success

I told you it wasn't complicated, but that doesn't mean it's not effective. In fact, you can use it as a framework to evaluate the weight-loss claims of any program and to guide your own lifestyle to a healthier place. The best part is that, candidly, you don't have to be part of the LadyBoss community to use it. It will work no matter who uses it. I just want to see you succeed. So let me break it down for you.

(**Fitness + Nutrition**) x Accountability = Success

If you want a healthy lifestyle that includes weight-loss, *fitness* and *nutrition* are like *love* and *marriage*. According to the old song, you can't have one without the other if you want to succeed.

The funny thing is that most weight-loss programs tell you that you can split the two up and still do just fine. They emphasize one and barely mention the other in the fine print. Some nutrition-focused diets even go so far as to claim you don't have to exercise at all. Other fitness-focused programs claim you can eat pretty much whatever you want, as long as you live in the gym. Both extremes are nonsense. You need to both eat healthy and act healthy.

Fitness is about what you do with your body, living an active life with a structured workout and exercise routine. You don't have to become a bodybuilder to learn your way around the gym or home fitness equipment. But you will have to do the hard work of exercising, pushing past your comfort zone to take your physical health to the next level.

Nutrition is about what you put into your body, eating and drinking in ways that position you to be the very best version of you. You don't have to become a dietician to learn the best foods that give you the best energy. But you will have to discipline yourself to say *yes* to the good and *no* to the bad, especially when trying to break old habits and establish new ones. And that's where the third and most important part of the Formula comes in.

(Fitness + Nutrition) x **Accountability** = Success

You may remember from algebra class in school that whatever is in parentheses ( ) gets done first. What's in parentheses is the most basic part of any formula. In the LadyBoss Formula, Fitness and Nutrition are the two fundamental components because they are in parentheses.

And it doesn't matter which one comes first for you. The best place to start is with whichever one is easiest to inject into your current lifestyle. If it's easier or more exciting for you to start with one or the other, that's fine. If you're more excited about working out than prepping meals, get to the gym. If you're more interested at first in learning how to eat better, start cooking up nutritious meals. In other words, don't wait to do both. Start where you are and work your way forward.

Because Fitness and Nutrition are both equally essential, the LadyBoss Formula shows them as being interchangeable. However, the third component Accountability functions in a different way. Accountability increases the effect of Fitness and Nutrition and *multiplies* their impact exponentially. If there were a secret to weight-loss and healthier living, it would be Accountability.

I discovered the power of Accountability by accident really. Certainly, as an athlete I knew the power of being part of a team. I knew how feeling accountable to my team members made me try harder on the basketball court, because I had to face them in the huddle afterwards. After I committed to losing weight, though, I was alone at college. I had zero accountability, and probably very little chance of success. Without even giving it much thought, I did something that I know made all the difference—I shared my commitment and journey on social media.

Suddenly, I began to hear from total strangers following my journey and encouraging me to keep my commitment. They reminded me of how special I really was. They showed me I had a responsibility that was bigger than myself. They let me know *my* journey was an encouragement to *them*—I never saw that coming, but it soon became a huge part of my motivation.

It's just too easy to think you are all alone on this journey to take control of your weight and live a healthy life. When your muscles ache after the first few weeks of a new workout routine, you start thinking you can skip a session, because no one will ever know. When you've had a bad day and the ice cream starts calling your name, you tell yourself no one will care if you let your healthy habits slip a little. In fact, the people closest to you might even cheer when you stumble and fall. That's why we all need positive accountability.

I'm so privileged now to be part of the LadyBoss community. Frankly, I got the ball rolling, but all the awesome ladies in the community are really the ones who make the magic happen. They encourage me and each other to keep moving forward each and every day. We celebrate wins together, tell each other how awesome we truly are, and show some tough love when needed.

Microwaveable veggie packs are the easiest, most convenient way to get your greens in! Steamables are a great brand you can buy in the freezer section of any Wal-mart.

As I mentioned earlier, you do not have to join the LadyBoss community to benefit from the LadyBoss Formula. You do need to find a supportive community of your own to encourage you to take your healthy living success to the next level. You will need it on those days when you just don't feel like working out. You don't need to be an extrovert, either, to harness the incredible power of a community. But you do need to know you are not alone and that your accountability group will kick you in the butt when you feel like coasting or quitting.

Make the LadyBoss Formula the basic framework for your healthy living journey and you'll soon by celebrating your own success. How do I know? Because I hear the stories from women who've done it—and are doing it—every single day.

Someday soon, I want to hear your story too.

What's Holding You Back?

- If *fitness* and *nutrition* are like love and marriage, how are you doing at both? Are you doing well in one, but not-so-great with the other? Are you adding the two together or is one subtracting from the other? Rate yourself on the two scales below with a 10 being "I am totally on it!" and 1 being "Not even thinking about it."

  Fitness: 1   2   3   4   5   6   7   8   9   10
  Nutrition: 1   2   3   4   5   6   7   8   9   10

  Which one needs the most attention right now and what will you do about it? Remember to start where you are and work your way forward.

  _____

  _____

- Accountability increases the effect of Fitness and Nutrition and *multiplies* their impact exponentially. So what does your support network look like? Are you surrounded by encouragers or discouragers? List the names of other women you have enlisted or will enlist to be part of your accountability group:

If you could use some encouragement and accountability, visit LadyBoss.com to connect with more awesome ladies like yourself on the journey to a healthier life.

Chapter 7

5 Essential Steps for Success

You can do this! Are you feeling it? Now that you know the LadyBoss Formula for healthy living, you have the basic framework for success in place.

Before I debunk the lies you'll encounter and give you the truths you should embrace instead, it's time for some straight-talk about essential steps you'll need to take if you're serious about applying everything you learn along the way. I'm going to put on my LadyBoss coaching hat in this chapter and really get candid with you. I don't want you to miss out on success when you're *so close* to putting all the pieces together.

If you're ready to get real and experience real weight-loss success, then let's do this! Here are five essential steps for weight-loss success based on my own success and the support I provide thousands of woman who are part of the LadyBoss movement:

Visit freecravingscheatsheet.com to download my free Cheat Sheet on how to crush the cravings that are holding you back from losing the weight!

1. Win the Battle in Your Mind

You are already a *freaking winner*! If you're still reading, you've probably already done the hardest part by admitting you need to change. You've made the mental shift and decided you need to do something different. That makes you a winner already. Sure, there will be challenging moments ahead, but you humbled yourself enough to do something different. That decision is *huge* because most of the battle ahead will be lost or won in your own mind.

So what are you thinking? The battle to lose weight and realize a healthy lifestyle is not an information battle, although you *will* learn a lot. It's not primarily a physical battle, even though it *will* involve fitness and nutrition. It's a battle inside your own mind to overcome the thoughts that don't align with your goals.

It's true for fitness. You have to learn how to mentally prepare yourself and tell yourself every day that you can do it. It's not doing the cardio workout or the weight training that's hard. What's hard is making the decision to get off the couch and go to the gym when you could watch a movie and eat popcorn in your cozy house.

The same is true for nutrition. When you're trying to eat healthy foods, it's the decision you make between seeing something and eating something that makes all the difference. When one side of your brain says, *That cheeseburger looks really, really good*, you can still win when the other side chooses the grilled chicken salad. Making the healthy choice is the hardest part. But if you know that the battle begins in your mind, you can prepare to fight there first.

One of the tricks I use is to allow myself a cheat meal once each week. That's how I could lose 65 pounds without giving up pizza and ice cream. You can designate one meal each week to enjoy your favorite foods as they should be enjoyed. If you know you can enjoy pizza on Saturday, it's easier to say no to pizza on Tuesday. Just procrastinate your enjoyment to a guilt-free time that fits within your plan. The truth is that letting yourself enjoy one cheat meal each week is good for your body's metabolism, a point I'll explain more later.

You must tell yourself you want long-term success more than the short-term enjoyment of the Reese's Cup in front of you. You must call out those moments of temptation and know what your body's trying to do to you. Then choose to take control of your body rather than letting it control you. Choose to do what's good for your body instead of what tastes good or what will feel good in the moment. Get yourself in that winning mindset. Be prepared. Be mentally strong and let's do this!

Let's face it, a lot of your weight-loss success will be determined by your attitude! Your attitude is the only thing in life you can control 100% of the time. You can't always control what's happening in your daily, crazy life. You can't control what other people are saying or what they're doing, but you can control your attitude.

I think of it as my attitude bubble. Inside my bubble is what I can control. All the other stuff out there may concern me, but I can't do much about it. No matter what's happening or going wrong out there, I know that I get to choose what my attitude is like in here. I get to choose to have a happy day. I get to choose to be excited about life and be the personality I enjoy being. Whenever I feel myself reacting to something, getting angry or frustrated, I tell myself, *Nope! I have 100% control of how I respond. I might not have control over the person who just wrecked my car or family drama going on, but I can control my attitude.*

One final tip for maintaining the right mindset is to compare the challenge you face in the moment to one you already overcame in the past. When it gets hard to work out one day, think about how it isn't hard to do compared to your first week or that first round of cardio you survived. Compare it to things you've already overcome and realize you don't even want the donuts someone just brought in. You don't even want that chocolate cake, because you've already made it through harder stuff and you can overcome this.

Remember you are *already a winner* for choosing to change. You keep winning each day when you focus on winning the battle in your own mind. You can do it! I'm already so proud of you!!

2. Change Your Story

The next step to experiencing lasting lifestyle change is to change your story. For me, the negative story I told myself every day was that I was overweight and out of shape for all the following reasons:

I'm lazy.

I just don't have enough energy.

It runs in my family.

No one around me is healthy.

I have a food addiction, so there's nothing I can do about it.

That was the story I told myself, *until* I decided to change my story. Instead of mindlessly repeating that failed plot line, I decided I would *not* let those things define me. I chose to rewrite my story to become an awesome, healthy, and energetic person who goes to the gym every day and inspires other people to live healthier lives. Once I changed the story I was telling myself every day, my mind and body followed. Stop telling yourself a negative story based on your past struggles. You can choose to rewrite your story, too.

First, you have to get disgusted with normal. Whatever *normal* is for you, it clearly isn't working right? But until it disgusts you, you'll tend to let it hang around. So many people settle for average, but you are better than that! Don't shoot for average.

Set a scary goal that will challenge you to push yourself. When I weighed 180 pounds, I really didn't think I was ever going to step onstage anywhere, but I pushed myself to reach for that level of success. The growth zone is never comfortable, but there's no growth in the comfort zone. Getting disgusted with normal and setting a lofty goal made me push myself out of my comfort zone.

What's a scary goal for you? Losing a hundred pounds? Getting to 9% body fat? Getting back into your high school jeans? Whatever seems scary to you, it's a lot more realistic than you think. I work with ladies all the time who are surprised at how quickly success happens when chasing a scary goal. Even if you miss a goal that seems unrealistic to you, you're going to end up a lot farther ahead than if you had set an average goal. When you settle for *average*, you don't really push yourself. Don't shoot for average, and you *will* surprise yourself.

Second, you change your story by, not surprisingly, telling yourself a different story in your own mind. Instead of telling yourself a story of failure and helplessness, tell yourself awesome things about you. Start telling yourself you want to do what you're currently doing, not what you've done in the past. Don't go back there. That's why the rearview mirror is a lot smaller than the windshield. Look forward, and tell yourself what you're going to do, instead of things you've failed to do in the past.

Finally, say positive things out loud to yourself all day long. One of my favorites is saying, *I'm awesome! I look good in this outfit and I'm happy because I'm healthy!!* Tell yourself the truth: *I'm awesome and full of energy. I consistently work out and pursue my goals. I eat healthy and I feel amazing!* Even if you don't fully believe the things you're saying to yourself yet, you will make yourself begin to believe them.

Once you start looking in the mirror and literally telling yourself those things, you'll start rewriting the story in your own mind. You have to give yourself those positive affirmations, because in today's world, we don't have many people who will tell us those truths on a regular basis. Give yourself credit for the things that you do and love yourself more.

3. Follow Your Proven Game Plan

Can I just be super honest with you? Anyone who tells you that it will be easy achieving your weight-loss and healthy living goals is lying to you. It is going to hurt sometimes. Any program that tells you otherwise is just stealing your money.

The hardest part is following a proven game plan to develop new habits. Until you get used to your body being in motion again, it's going to hurt—but that's what you want. You want it to hurt, so you can overcome it and get results that fit your new story. If your body isn't sore at all when starting a new fitness routine, then you're not pushing yourself enough. I'm going to tell you straight up, expect your body to be sore. Expect to feel the burn. That's ok. That's how you know you're working hard and pushing your body toward success.

The mistake I tended to make early on was stopping too soon. Instead of doing 15 reps, I would stop at 10. Instead of doing 30 minutes of cardio, I would stop at 20. But I was only hurting myself. Don't be that woman! If you have a plan to do 30 minutes, do it! Push through the resistance. Block out what your mind is telling you, because your body will keep going. It's the final reps and those additional minutes that are the most important.

Sure, it's going to hurt, but it's going to be worth it if you don't quit. That's why I started LadyBoss, to give women like you a proven plan to succeed, complete with exercise routines, healthy meal options, and plenty of encouragement. I don't want you to have an excuse to quit!

You are so close to realizing your healthy lifestyle dreams *if you don't quit!* It's finally within your grasp, but that doesn't mean it's convenient. It's never going to be convenient to lose weight, build muscle, eat healthy, or completely change your lifestyle. It's never going to be convenient, but there are plenty of other things in your life that aren't convenient that you do. Paying bills isn't convenient for me every month, I can tell you that. But I do it anyways. Paying taxes, making sure kids get picked up on time, or having to stay at work late— none of these things are convenient, but we do them anyways. Why? Because the lasting consequences for not doing them far outweighs the temporary inconvenience.

That's the mindset you have to have when it comes to following your proven plan. Whether it be the LadyBoss Lifestyle Program or your own healthy living lifestyle built on the truths I'll unpack in the next chapters, it will all come down to you actually doing what needs to be done *no matter what*. When it gets challenging, push through the resistance and do it anyway.

Don't quit on yourself again this year. How many years now have you been saying, "I'm going to lose this twenty pounds," or, "I'm going to lose the baby weight?" How long has it been? You cannot quit on yourself. You *cannot* quit on what you could do for your kids, and your family, and the person that you could be, and the confidence that you could have.

I know it's really easy to get off track and think there will be a better time to get serious about losing weight. But there's never a good time. It's never convenient. There will always be other stuff you have to do. You have to make time for it now. Trust me, the time is going to pass anyway. *This* is the moment when you need to buckle down, say, "I'm going to do it anyway. It's not convenient, but I'm going to make time for it, and I can do this." I believe in you! You're *not* a quitter, and I'm not going to let you become one!!

I don't expect you to do everything every single day, but you do need to be aware of where you're being most consistent. None of the members of the LadyBoss movement ever do every single workout, follow every meal plan exactly, or plug in to every single chat group and watch every video. It's just not possible. Life happens.

Start where you are, but don't stay there. If you naturally do well with nutrition and meal plans, for example, be intentional about getting your fitness routines up to speed as quickly as possible. If fitness is a natural fit for you, start there but be intentional about getting your nutrition and meal plans in place. Don't let your desire to get it perfect stop you from starting. But keep striving to be better in all areas—fitness, nutrition and accountability.

4. Embrace the Law of Results

If you're going to resist temptation and stay on course, you'll need to embrace the law of results. Results don't just happen; you must consistently do the actions required to achieve the results you want. That's how the law works: if you do the work, you'll see the results.

Excuses won't cut it. You can either have excuses or have results. You can achieve your goals, or you can you have the excuses, but you can't have both. You have to be consistent. Consistency is key. It's a battle we all have to fight every single day. Here's how to follow through when you're tempted to drop out.

First, realize you're *not* perfect. None of us are psychologically or emotionally perfect beings; we're all going to crave certain foods at times. Whether you're a chocolate person, a savory person, or a salty person, you're going to have those cravings that can trip you up. Realize that your body is going to crave these things and develop an awareness of what your body wants.

Second, prepare for the craving by knowing a healthy alternative. If your body is craving chocolate, for example, maybe whip up one of the chocolate mud cakes in the LadyBoss Lifestyle Program. If your body's craving something savory, look for something that's savory but healthy. Instead of reaching for a bag of potato chips, make zucchini chips instead. Find the healthier alternative and—most importantly—have it ready when the craving comes.

Third, know that you will see temptation everywhere you go. The grocery store, gas station, vending machines—you name it, temptation is out there. The key is to understand that *you* are in control of it. The Hershey bar does not control you. The Doritos do not control you. You're in charge of you. You are writing your own story. You need to be in control of those cravings so you can achieve the results you want.

5. Stay Connected to a Community

Accountability is the force multiplier in the LadyBoss Formula. (Fitness + Nutrition) x Accountability = Success. It's the secret sauce, if you will, that releases the power of fitness and nutrition. So many of us women think we are alone in the struggle to lose weight and live healthier lives. It's not true. We're all in this together.

You don't have to be part of the LadyBoss community to find that support, but you do need support. You need to be connected to an encouraging community that will inspire you to keep moving forward and give you a kick in the butt on those days when you feel like quitting.

The community needs you as much as you need the community. You bring something unique to any group. Your consistent efforts in pursuit of your dream will inspire other women in your community. They need you to inspire *them* as much as you need them to inspire and encourage *you*. That's why it's critical that you go public with your journey and document your efforts. You need people who can cheer you on for making it to the gym four times this week or for saying *no* to that decadent, chocolate dessert last night.

Remember, if you're consistent with anything, you're pretty much lapping the people still sitting on the couch. Even if you're just making consciously healthy food choices or simply being consistent in getting to the gym, you're inspiring other people to get off the couch and do something different. Stay consistent. Do it for the community of people around you, and they will be there for you when you need that same encouragement.

A supportive group like the LadyBoss community can help you get *unstuck*. When you think, *Oh my gosh, I would love to sit here and eat an entire tub of ice cream*, you can share that feeling with your community so they can remind you of your goals. They can help you focus on the dream you're achieving later, instead of the craving you're feeling right now. They can help you remember your *why* and keep it in front of you when the going gets tough.

You need friends who will support you, not discourage you so they will feel better about their own failures. Your community can help you celebrate victories together. No matter how big or small they are, telling your friends makes the victories feel more real. Post your victories on Facebook and Instagram and celebrate each and every step of success—both yours and theirs. I love celebrating all the wins of the ladies in the LadyBoss community and look forward to reading about all the victories they share.

Sometimes we can trick ourselves into not sharing about success, because we don't want anyone else to feel bad or think we're bragging. But you can't be afraid of those things. Whether it's losing a pound or an inch, or just making it to the 20-minute

Purge bad foods from your home. Clean out your cabinets and pantries of all trigger foods and replace with healthy options to snack on!

mark running on the treadmill—whatever it is, don't be afraid to tell the world about it.

Bottom line: Find a community that will celebrate your wins with you. I'd love to connect with you and be there to cheer you on as a part of the LadyBoss community. You can find out more about our community at LadyBoss.com.

But wherever you get plugged in, connect with a community as you live out these five essential steps and put the LadyBoss Formula to work to achieve your dreams. You are not alone and deserve support every step of the way. YOU. ARE. AWESOME!

What's Holding You Back?

- Think about your own *attitude bubble*. Do you think about yourself as being in control or do your cravings control you? What do you choose to think about yourself each day? How seriously do you take the battle in your own mind? Take some time to describe the positive attitude you want to have about your weight-loss journey.

  _____

  _____

  _____

- It's time to start changing your story. Most women don't give themselves enough credit for being beautiful and amazing people. The more you start telling yourself how amazing you really are, the more you're going to let your true light shine. I can't wait for you to know how awesome that feels. On the lines below, start rewriting your story with "I am awesome, because ..."

_____

_____

_____

- What's your proven game plan? Do you have one? Go ahead and take the time to outline your strategy for weight-loss success below. If you don't have one, I encourage you to visit LadyBoss.com where you can get access to the LadyBoss Weight-loss Program.

_____

_____

_____

- Do you have a plan for dealing with cravings? List the cravings you tend to have and at least three healthy alternatives for each. You may need to do some research online or in the LadyBoss Program to find better choices. Once you find them, have them ready so you can overcome temptation and make healthier choices.

_____

_____

_____

- Do you feel alone? If you have a supportive community that encourages you and holds you accountable, take a moment to list their names below. Then send them a note, an email, or social message thanking them for their support.

_____

_____

_____

LadyBoss Success Story

Macil Melton, Huntington, WV

I've struggled with my weight since having my first child, I was 280 lbs. at my heaviest. Through on and off dieting, I got down to about 230 lbs. I had tried all the fad diets, water pills, laxatives and shakes and nothing worked. All the money was just wasted on things I didn't see quick results from. I was always tired, had no energy to do anything, and ate out of pure boredom. I hated pictures and would always try to be the one taking them every chance I got.

In 2012, my life was flipped upside down. My husband and childhood sweetheart was diagnosed with brain cancer. He had been healthy his whole life, and he gets handed a death sentence while there I sat—overweight and unhealthy. He was stricken with something out of his control, and there I was, slowly killing myself.

In 2013, I decided enough was enough. I cleaned my eating up and started working out daily. Though the weight was dropping, it was dropping too fast, and I still found myself tired, even worse than before. I had gone from one extreme to the other. I went from eating anything and everything to restricting my calories to under 900 and working out 3 hours a day. I had also tried purging by this point.

So, I reevaluated everything yet again, did some research, and started eating appropriately and working out for 1.5-2 hrs. a day.

I've completed several 5ks, 10ks, and 3 half marathons, as well as receiving my certification in personal training. My husband died Dec 3, 2015. I had lost my way and gained 20 lbs. back when I saw Kaelin's video come across my newsfeed. Something just spoke to me, motivated me, and that drive I once had came flooding back. I really thought I'd never get that part of me back after losing my husband until I saw her and watched her video.

I've been in the LadyBoss movement for about a month now, hardcore for about 3 weeks. I don't weigh myself, but my clothes are fitting better; I feel amazing, and my BF/BMI percentages have already dropped. I have more confidence after joining the LadyBoss movement. I feel stronger both physically and emotionally, and I just can't thank Kaelin enough!

Chapter 8

Weight-Loss Lies

Big Fat Lie #1

You can't lose weight without giving up the foods you love.

The Truth:

You can still enjoy the foods you love while losing weight.

When most people think of a healthy lifestyle, they think they have to give up the foods they love and eat broccoli for the rest of their lives. Not true.

I lost 65 pounds and got into great shape while still enjoying pizza and ice cream every single week. How? By planning a "cheat meal" into every week. I mentioned this trick earlier, but almost every Saturday night I get to enjoy my favorite pizza and Coldstone cake-batter ice cream. My eyes are always bigger than my stomach, so I usually look forward to eating an entire pizza on Saturday night then feel full after just one piece.

A weekly cheat meal—not an entire cheat day—keeps you sane. When you're eating healthy and staying fit, you'll often think about those favorite foods, especially when stressed out. But knowing you will enjoy them at a single designated time empowers you to resist the urge to splurge. Treat it as a reward. If you stick to your plan all week, you can enjoy your cheat meal guilt-free!

I'm not just offering this cheat meal idea to make you feel better psychologically about eating foods you love. There's actual science behind it. Your body needs it. I discovered this fact when training for the body-building competition. When your body is eating healthy foods all week—salads, veggies, and lean proteins—your metabolism doesn't have to work very hard to digest and metabolize those healthy foods. A cheat meal

Choose a smaller plate. Science shows that the plate you choose to eat from influences how much you put on it. Switch to a smaller plate, and you could reduce your calorie intake by 20 percent!

really ramps up your metabolism and reinvigorates your digestive system. Because pizza, hamburgers, donuts, ice cream, or *whatever* you can dream of requires more energy to digest, your body reacts by turning up your metabolism, which actually gets your next week off to a great start.

Now, don't get me wrong. We're talking about one meal, an entrée and a dessert, eaten in one sitting, not an entire buffet of treats spread out over several nights. Used wisely, a cheat meal will help you make progress physically and mentally toward your goal.

The other way to still enjoy foods you love is to satisfy your cravings with healthy alternatives. Most people just don't know about all the ways to substitute healthier foods and still enjoy the same great tastes. And healthier options do not have to be super expensive.

What I did in the beginning of my weight-loss journey was to list out my favorite trigger foods. Chocolate, pizza, and burgers are all trigger foods for me. At that point in my life, anytime I would hear the word *burger* or *pizza* I would give in. The craving is what it is; I had to learn how to satisfy that craving in a healthy way. Instead of avoiding the cravings, I found alternatives that taste just like what I wanted. I make pizza myself out of cauliflower crust, turkey pepperonis, fat-free cheese, and marinara sauce. Now I really can't even tell the difference in satisfying a craving with healthy pizza or typical pizza. The reality is that you're always gong to fail in the moment of craving if you don't prepare healthy alternatives beforehand.

I wrote down my trigger foods then researched healthy alternatives, something I challenge you to do on the next pages. More and more grocery stores carry these healthier options. Here are a few examples of foods I crave and the healthy alternatives I discovered:

- **Ice Cream**

  Halo Top or Arctic Zero ice cream, protein ice creams with only a couple hundred calories per pint. You can also literally make ice cream out of a protein shake or shave ice to make a snow cone and top it with a tasty Mio flavor.

- **Gatorade, Energy Drinks, and Soda**

  A lot of these drinks have way too many calories and too much sugar. I use Mio instead to create a healthier alternative. Sometimes I add it to carbonated water to get a healthy drink that satisfies my soda cravings.

- **Chocolate or Sweets**

  Quest bars are my healthy alternative of choice when the sweet craving hits (White chocolate is one of my trigger foods, so I have to be ready.) Quest bars come in dozens of flavors, including chocolate, s'mores, cookie dough, brownie—you name it.

  Sugar-free Jell-O is another of my favorite alternatives. It satisfies the craving and fills me up without adding calories and pounds. Terrific late-night snack!

- **Fried Foods**

  I use Almond Flour as a healthy alternative to breading. I make jalapeno poppers by filling little egg "cups" in a mini-muffin pan with peppers and fat-free cheese. Once baked, I get cute little egg poppers to dip in salsa. They are SO good!

- **Salty Snacks**

  Speaking of salsa, it's good for you. Try dipping in some Nut-Thins if you like crunchy snacks. Zucchini chips also make a great alternative to potato chips and Doritos. I make them almost every day. Just cut them up really thin, broil them in the oven, and put some garlic seasoning on top.

- **Pasta**

  Pasta Zero is a zero-carb pasta that lets you enjoy pasta once again while still eating healthy.

- **Coffee**

  A lot of us love coffee, but what we put into it can make weight-loss difficult. I use Stevia as a sweetener, because it comes from a natural monk fruit. My favorite drink at Starbucks is a cold brew, with almond milk, sugar-free caramel, and three Stevia. It's an iced coffee and SO good!

Discover more ideas within the LadyBoss Lifestyle Program or by reviewing my social media sites for videos on alternatives. The important thing is knowing that cravings will come—and being prepared to control them.

Make your own chips by broiling zucchini slices in the oven for 5-10 minutes until crispy. Put garlic seasoning for taste!

Big Fat Lie #2

You have to count calories and eat less to lose weight.

The Truth:

All calories are not created equal, and you must eat more to lose more.

Mind-blowing, I know. Ever since the 1,000-calorie diet became popular years ago, women have thought calorie count is key to losing weight. So they starve themselves to consume as few calories as possible. What they don't realize is not all calories are created equal. 1,000 calories of Oreos and cheese is not the same as 1,000 calories of vegetables and lean proteins—the stuff that actually fuels the body.

What makes the difference is not the number of macronutrients—protein, fat, or carbs—but the quality of the micronutrients— the real ingredients in the food. Because micronutrients determine whether or not your body can use the food as fuel. There is no magic number that you must hit to lose weight. It's all about ensuring your calories, proteins, fats, and carbs are coming from healthy sources—lean proteins, healthy fats, and complex carbs. If you're eating foods from those three groups, you can eat as much as you want. You can eat until you're full because it's not about *how much* you eat, it's about *what* you're eating.

This fear of eating too much causes women to believe the lie that they have to eat less to lose weight. Just the opposite is true. Your body is like a caveman trying to survive. If you go without food because you're counting calories, your body's going to hold onto the fat, and the carbs, and all the things that you want it to burn, because it doesn't know when it's going to get the next meal. It's a natural defense mechanism of your body to hold on to whatever it gets when you skip meals and don't eat enough. You actually just need to eat more of the right things to let your body move past the caveman survival thinking.

Understand that food is *fuel.* Every time you eat ask, *Is this fueling my body for a purpose?* If the answer is *yes,*

Don't eat in front of the TV or computer. This triggers mindless eating and causes you to over eat. So turn off the TV & focus on your meal.

then you can eat as much as you want. You're not going to get fat by eating green vegetables. To lose weight, eat every two to three hours. Have breakfast when you wake up, then have a snack about three hours later. Eat lunch, have an afternoon snack, then dinner and another snack later at night. You want to keep your metabolism running consistently and burning good fuel, not starving and storing fat.

Your metabolism is basically like a campfire. When a campfire starts dying out, we put on more logs as fuel for the fire. Our metabolism is the same. When our metabolism starts slowing down every three hours or so, we should put more logs on. It speeds our metabolism back up and keeps it burning calories for us all day long. It's much more important to keep your body fueled and your metabolism moving than it is to care about how many calories you're getting, especially if you're uniting nutrition with fitness and staying active.

When you put healthy foods on your metabolism fire, the flames will burn well and take everything with it. Keep eating the wrong stuff, and it won't burn well at all. That's how the fat builds up. Instead of starving yourself, keep your body fueled consistently with more healthy food.

A sweet Protein/Nutrition shake will help curb your sweet cravings late at night. At LadyBossLabs. com we have the best-tasting shake in the world specifically formulated for women.

Big Fat Lie #3

You can't go out to eat and still lose weight.

The Truth:

You can go out
to eat and still
lose weight IF
you make good
choices.

I used to believe this lie. One of my favorite things to do is to share some quality time with people as we gather around a meal. I didn't want to give it up to lose weight. I thought I had to—but I was wrong.

So many women think they have to give up everything they love, including having dinner with friends and family. Don't get me wrong, you do have to make sacrifices to live a healthy lifestyle that will empower you to fulfill your dreams. But you don't have to give up everything and definitely not eating out.

The last thing you need when trying to lose weight is to feel isolated and alone. I remember being the only one at the table with chicken and a salad when I was first trying to lose weight. People get afraid of going out to lunch with their co-workers because they don't know what to order and feel embarrassed. Society makes you feel guilty now if you're the one eating healthy. I don't want you to feel like you can't go out to eat; you need healthy relationships for a healthy life.

You have to learn how to order the food that you enjoy *without* all the extra junk that makes it unhealthy. That means ordering chicken in the restaurant but asking them to hold the butter and oil. Order an Italian dish like chicken marsala, but get the sauce on the side and leave the mushrooms. It comes down to making wise choices. You really can't take a huge pasta dish and make it healthy, but you can start with a healthy base like salmon and a baked potato with no butter and sour cream.

The key to success when dining out is to decide what you will order before you go. It's never been easier with so many restaurants now offering online menus you can view in advance. Once you're there and hungry, it becomes harder to make

Replace dessert with fresh fruit. It's a better way to satisfy your sweet tooth & most restaurants offer it as a dessert as well.

smart choices about what to eat. Look up the menu before you go—when you're not hungry or feeling pressured by your friends to make an unhealthy decision.

To be honest, I struggled with this for the longest time. When I got to the restaurant, I would have this battle in my own mind that went something like: *I know I should order the tilapia with mango salsa, but this big, huge pasta dish with all the sauce and sausage looks really good.* Once I realized I was usually losing that battle, I made my choice before I went. Now I regularly enjoy going out to eat without being worried about gaining weight.

One word of warning: don't try to pressure your friends and family into following your example. If they ask why you chose the food you did, tell them you've made a decision to make healthier lifestyle choices. But don't scold them for choosing pizza and wings while you chose something healthier.

The way you get them to join you is not by shaming them for what they're eating. Let's face it. You used to do the same thing, and the last thing you wanted was to be guilt-tripped into eating healthy. Let your results speak for themselves. Then when other people want help on their own journey, they'll come to you.

You have to realize this is the path that you have chosen; this is the choice that you have made. Other people around you haven't made that choice yet. You can't force it on them. If you do, that's when you *will* become isolated. Lead by example, and they'll come to you for advice when they're ready.

Save hundreds of calories by getting your dressing on the side and dipping your fork in for each bite!

Big Fat Lie #4

You're only having success if your scale's going down.

The Truth:

Your scale is a liar. Throw it out now.

You should throw your freaking bathroom scale away. No, seriously. As soon as you finish reading this section, go chuck it in the trash. It's worse than worthless, because it's lying to you. It's telling you numbers that have very little to do with how healthy you are—but most women think they're the only numbers that matter.

Once again, the weight-loss industry has set you up to fail by pushing the lie that dropping pounds is how you should measure success. This way they can sell you programs that deliver immediate weight-loss results. The fact that you'll put those pounds right back on—and then some—doesn't matter to them. The fact that losing weight the wrong way can actually make you unhealthy doesn't matter to them.

I care more about your living a healthy life than your buying products and programs, so I'm just going to shoot straight with you—THROW OUT YOUR SCALE!

Women like you get up every single day, weigh themselves, and get so discouraged they don't follow through on their healthy living game plan. They take one look at the numbers on the scale and get so depressed they quit before they begin. Weighing yourself first thing in the morning is like starting your day by lighting yourself on fire, rolling around in broken glass, and then throwing yourself off a cliff. That's how it feels when you think you're making progress doing the right things but the scale says you've actually gained three pounds. Am I right?

Listen to me—a gallon of water weighs eight pounds. If you're drinking a gallon of water a day—like you should be doing—your weight can vary a lot depending on how

Halo Top & Arctic Zero are great healthy alternatives to ice cream! They taste amazing and you can eat a serving guilt free!

much is still inside you. I've known women who actually stop drinking enough water so the scale will tell them they're making progress. It doesn't work that way. Drink what you should and toss the scale. It will always mislead you.

The biggest reason your scale can't help you measure success is that the scale can't tell the difference between muscle and fat. Muscle is denser than fat, but the scale doesn't read your body composition. It doesn't know the difference. The Body Mass Index (BMI) has the same problem. According to the BMI scale I am actually "obese" right now, even though I am in the best shape of my life and healthy as can be. So ignore that, too. In the LadyBoss community, we stress body fat percentage and inches lost to measure your success. Every other popular measurement doesn't tell you what you really want to know.

Muscle gives you the shape and the figure you really want. What you see in models and actors whose bodies you admire is muscle definition. When you're building that *muscle definition* you're building denser tissue. That denser muscle tissue is going to take up less space. That's why in my LadyBoss program we emphasize measuring *inches* lost more than pounds lost. The inches women in the LadyBoss community lose are crazy!

Unless they are very overweight, they may lose only ten pounds, but drop thirty inches overall—and they look GREAT! They look like they lost fifty pounds and they're healthy as can be, because they're ignoring the scale and focusing on getting *leaner*, not *lighter*.

We have had a lot of women in the LadyBoss program for three months who haven't lost a single pound, and yet they've lost twenty inches! Which would you rather have—a scale in your bathroom that says you lost ten pounds, or the whole world being able to see that you've dropped five pant sizes in three months?

If you want more visual proof, look at the pictures of me below. I weigh exactly the same in both photos. Hard to believe isn't it! If

I went by the scale, I'd be discouraged in Photo #2 even though I look great. That's why I say the scale doesn't tell you what you need to know. It only discourages you from moving forward with your proven game plan.

The reality is that every body is different. Your weight is not a reliable indicator of your success. As you get leaner and build more muscle through strength training, your body fat percentage goes down. When that happens, your inches go down. Your muscle tone improves, and your body gets smaller and tighter. Your clothes fit better as your fat goes away, even if the scale says your weight isn't dropping drastically.

So quit discouraging yourself and putting seeds of doubt in you mind by getting on the scale every day. It's the wrong measuring stick. Throw. It. Out. NOW!

137 POUNDS

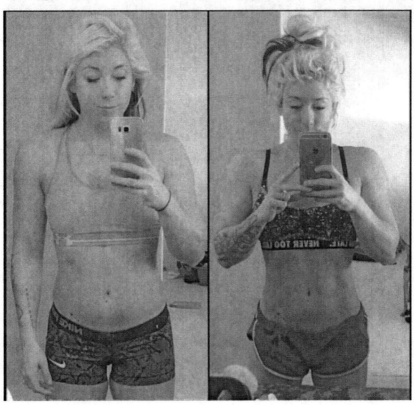

Big Fat Lie #5

Weight-loss should happen on a specific timeline.

The Truth:

Everyone's weight-loss timeline is different.

When most women set out to lose weight, they immediately give themselves a deadline, a specific timeline to measure success. Maybe they ask a friend how long it took her to lose weight. When the friend says she dropped the weight in three months, then that's the new deadline.

Right from the start, they're comparing themselves to someone else who has a completely different body and lifestyle. Does the friend have kids? Does she work full-time? Does she have the same body composition? Who knows! But three months is now the magical timeline for losing 30 pounds.

And when they only lose five pounds in the first month, they figure there's no way they can lose twenty-five pounds in two months, so why bother? They stop trying to lose weight and live a healthy life because they aren't seeing results as quickly as they think they should. More than likely, they'll wind up blaming whatever program they were on and telling everyone how it didn't work when they tried it.

The reality is most women start with false expectation, comparing themselves with other women instead of focusing on living a healthy lifestyle over the long-term. They are trying to do what some other person did in the same amount of time, even though they are completely different people with their own unique circumstances and body compositions. Everyone's results should be different. Just because I lost 65 pounds in 7 months doesn't mean you will or should.

You are not a failure if you don't lose a certain amount of weight in a certain amount of time—like so-and-so did. It doesn't mean you did something wrong. It doesn't mean that you

> When weight training in the gym, EFFORT is the ultimate measure of success. Always strive to do as many reps as you can.

weren't as good. It just means your body is different and your life is different. It's going to happen differently for each woman. For example, I lose weight starting in my face. Weird, I know, but that's the point. First I lose it from my face, then my shoulders, then my butt, my legs, and finally from my stomach and lats.

Other women lose weight in their stomach first and their legs last. Everyone is different. You're setting yourself up for failure when you compare your life and your body to someone else and put their weight-loss timeline on your own journey. It's just not possible for two women to have the same journey. No two flowers bloom the same, but they are all beautiful.

Comparison that produces an artificial timeline is unhealthy. You should have weight-loss goals, but tying them to timeline expectations can be dangerous. Instead, I coach woman in the LadyBoss community to focus on what they do every day. If you're trying to lose 30 pounds, what are the habits you have to have in place every single day? Focus on that single day. Focus on eating three healthy meals and two healthy snacks that day, drinking a gallon of water, doing your affirmations, writing your goals, and working out. If you focus on doing those five things every single day, you'll win every day. Your progress will snowball, and soon your momentum will produce the results you want.

Instead of wearing yourself out by focusing on the amount you want to lose in a certain timeframe, focus on doing the basics each day. Master the short-term habits, and long-term success will come.

When I was trying to lose the 65 pounds, it seemed so far away. There were days when I thought it would take forever, so why bother? I grabbed a tub of ice cream and said, *Screw it! This is taking too long.* But when I focused on the daily routines, not only did I get the results I wanted, I blew past them and won day after day. Before long I had lost the weight and gained a healthy lifestyle. And you can, too. I believe in you!

Big Fat Lie #6

You can experience instant weight-loss results.

The Truth:

Lasting weight-loss success is all about delayed gratification.

You see it on television ads all the time: *In as little as five minutes a day, you can shed the pounds and get the body you've always dreamed of. Or just 15 minutes a day, twice a week and you'll be rid of those extra pounds.* They promise instant results—but nothing could be further from the truth. With weight-loss, there are never instant results. Ever.

Real, lasting weight-loss is all about delayed gratification. You're not going to see results tomorrow from the workout you do today. The healthy food you eat today isn't going to magically transform your body by tomorrow, next week, or even two weeks later. Your body will start letting go of the weight after you do the right things consistently for weeks at a time.

It takes four weeks of renewed routines before you'll notice a difference in your body. It'll take eight weeks for your friends to notice a difference in your body when you're losing weight. The promise of instant results has discouraged so many women from sticking to a plan. They think they should see results within the first week, two weeks, or even a month—and if they don't, something must be wrong. But making the move to a healthy lifestyle isn't going to show in your body next week. It's going to start showing weeks and months later— and it's going to make a lasting difference in your life.

Only by being consistent in your workout and healthy heating habits can you expect to see results in your body four to eight weeks from now. But that truth doesn't sell weight-loss plans by preying on the hopes and fears of ladies all over the world. So, the weight-loss industry lies to you and leaves you even more frustrated when their "instant" plan fails.

These days it seems there's an app for everything. But there is no shortcut to weight-loss. You can't outsource it. You can't have someone else exercise for you or eat healthy while you down fried Twinkies. You must do it yourself. There is no magic pill. You must put in the work. You must put in the effort. If you don't do it consistently, you won't get the results you want.

This whole idea of instant results or even two-week results is total B.S., because you're not even going to notice a difference in yourself within four weeks. We women quit so many things within the first couple weeks because we expect the instant results we were sold on television infomercials that offer instant results--guaranteed. Then we quit when we don't see instant result in the mirror. We don't go to the gym and do the work, yet we say "It's not working" when we look in the mirror and don't see a change.

Listen up, ladies! It takes faith. We must trust that when we follow the process of nutrition (eating healthy) plus fitness (working out), good things will happen. You will start seeing the results you want when you consistently do the freaking hard work. You can't hack weight-loss. If you don't put in the work, you won't get the reward— no matter what "instant results" they promised you.

LadyBoss Success Story

Tabby Nevin, Nothfield VT

To this day I will never forget the day I realized how obese and unhealthy I was. I was talking with friends (in middle school), when I happened to look over at my reflection in a mirror, and I almost dropped to the floor. I cried and cried.

I was always enabled. I remembered being 8-years-old, and I would be picked on. When I cried to my mom and she would always say, "It's only baby fat; it will go away!" and then I would brush it off.

I ate nothing but McDonald's and other fast food as a child because that's what was convenient for my mom. That day in middle school is the day I wanted to change, although being young, it was difficult to know how and where to begin. I could never keep up with the kids in my class. I always had to shop in the bigger sections at stores. But still it was brushed off. My grandma once said to me as I was looking at a two piece bathing suit, "Don't you think you're a little too heavy to wear something like that?"

That was the day I started dieting and doing crazy exercise routines. Let me put it this way: I have tried everything out there!

I came across Kaelin when I was trying a different program, and she inspired me so much she made me believe you can do whatever you put your mind to; you can sculpt your dream body by putting the work in. I was following her for a while, and then she came out with the app. That's when I told myself, my doctors, and my dietitians: I'm going to do this! I suffered from high blood pressure, borderline diabetes, and sleep apnea.

Since I have started following Kaelin, I've gone from 245 lbs. to 155 lbs. I didn't measure myself, but I know by what my clothes say that those numbers aren't lying! I have so much more energy, and my blood pressure is perfect!! Plus, no more medications— the gym is the only prescription I need for my depression!

Chapter 9
Nutrition Lies

Big Fat Lie #7

Carbs are bad and make you fat.

The Truth:

You need carbonydrates to be healthy, and not all carbs are bad.

Back in the 1990s, the weight-loss industry was all about getting rid of fats. For the last decade, the focus has been on cutting out carbs—carbs are bad because they make you fat. They've made a TON of money telling people to cut carbs out of their diets. The South Beach diet is one low-carb approach.

All these fad diets claim carbs are evil because they make you fat; it's simply not true. Like calories and fats, all carbs are not created equal. Your body needs carbs because carbs are energy. But there is a difference between simple carbs and complex carbs. Simple carbs are basically simple sugars—candy, white bread, starchy stuff, flour, chips, etc. Simple carbs spike insulin levels and cause the liver to go into survival mode, signaling your body to save, save, save.

Complex carbs come mostly from the ground—vegetables, sprouted grain, sweet potatoes, Ezekiel bread, beans, etc. (Yes, some people actually say eating veggies is bad. See the list of complex carbs on the following pages.) Complex carbs don't spike insulin levels at all and are used immediately by the body as energy, not stored for future use.

Unfortunately, the weight-loss industry has lumped all carbs together to give them a bad rap. The diet industry bashes carbs because they need an enemy. But their attack on complex carbs hurts the very people they claim to help. Dumping complex carbs from your diet *can* cause short-term weight-loss—the weight-loss industry knows you will see results—but it will also cause long-term weight gain—up to 3 or 4 times what you originally lost.

Drink a protein / nutritional shake after your workout to refuel your body and your muscles so they can burn fat for you for up to 3 days.

For example, when I quit eating carbs for about twelve weeks, my body started shutting itself down. My brain functions slowed noticeably. It took me four seconds to remember my name and phone number. I was sick. I was tired all the time. I never had any energy. I was *super* moody. Without complex carbs, I was basically running on empty.

Once I started putting complex carbs back into my diet, I gained 40 pounds in 6 weeks! Everyone thought I was pregnant! I ended up with gluten intolerance, because my body literally couldn't digest it anymore after I had put it in starvation mode.

Back to the caveman example from earlier: if you cut out a major food group, your body will store up fat to burn because it doesn't know the next time it's going to get energy. Carbs are the most available energy source that fuels your mind and body. The diet industry has sold this carbs-are-bad thinking because you lose weight in the short-term. But they don't show all the weight people gain back once they get off the unsustainable diet. You can't cut out food groups and live a healthy lifestyle. Your body needs all three—lean proteins, healthy fats, and complex carbs.

If you're feeling hungry and you've already eaten, chances are you're actually dehydrated! Your body can easily mistake thirst for hunger.

List of Complex Carbs that Can Be Eaten Every Day

(One serving at a time of course!)

- All-bran cereals
- Apples
- Artichokes
- Asparagus
- Bananas
- Beans
- Broccoli
- Brown bread
- Brown rice
- Brussels sprouts
- Buckwheat
- Buckwheat bread
- Cabbage
- Carrots
- Cassava
- Cauliflower
- Celery
- Chickpeas
- Cucumbers
- Eggplant
- Garbanzo beans
- Grapefruits
- High fiber breakfast cereals
- Kidney beans
- Lentils
- Lettuce
- Muesli
- Multi-grain bread
- Navy beans
- Oat bran cereal
- Oatmeal
- Okra
- Onions
- Oranges
- Other root vegetables
- Peas
- Pinto beans
- Plums
- Porridge oats
- Potato
- Prunes
- Radishes
- Shredded wheat
- Soybeans
- Spinach
- Split peas

- Sprouts
- Strawberries
- Sweet potato
- Tomatoes
- Turnip greens

- Watercress
- Weetabix
- Whole barley
- Whole grain cereals

- Whole grain flours
- Whole meal bread
- Wild rice
- Yam
- Zucchini

Big Fat Lie #8

Eating fats
makes you fat.

The Truth:

Eating fats makes you fit.

Most people think putting fats into their bodies will make them fat. But that's not necessarily true. Like carbs, not all fats are equal. If you're talking about *saturated* fats like butter, *then* eating saturated fats makes you fat. Saturated fats are bad. But eating healthy fats actually lets your body release stored fat.

Your body stores fat when it doesn't get the healthy fats it needs to survive. When your body gets the healthy fats it needs, it releases what it had stockpiled and replenishes with healthy fats. Healthy fats are like logs on the campfire, the long-burning fuel that gives our bodies the energy we need. Complex carbs are like the twigs and smaller branches that burn faster and brighter. Both types of fuel are needed for a fire to burn well. Our body needs both to sustain a healthy metabolism and burn energy cleanly and effectively.

The problem today is that we have so much processed food with very little nutritional value your body can actually use. Most of the fats in processed foods are saturated fats. Great sources of healthy fats include avocados, almond butter, nuts, fish, and coconut oil (I cook everything in it!).

The nutrition industry has used this lie about fats to sell products. Take a look at the shelves in your local grocery store, and you'll see labels claiming to be *non-fat* and *fat-free* as if having no fat means it's good for you. In reality, that product may just be loaded with sugar. They've portrayed fat as the enemy stuff. Just because their chips are *fat-free* doesn't mean they're not loaded with 100g of sugar, simple carbs your body will turn into unhealthy fat. Don't buy the lie and assume all fats are bad. Do your homework, and don't be fooled into thinking the *fat-free* label automatically means *healthy*.

Drink a glass of Lemon Water a day. It helps get rid of toxic waste in the body and detox your system.

Another good source of fat is grass-fed beef with a little bit of fat in it, or 93% lean ground turkey. The key is moderation and not going too crazy with fats, like eating an entire can of nuts, for example. Your body needs fats to burn as long-lasting fuel. That's why I love to start each day with almond butter on rice cakes to give my brain some fuel to start the day.

Big Fat Lie #9

It takes a lot of time to eat healthy.

The Truth:

Eating healthy takes less time, not more.

What a lie! For years I believed it takes a lot of time to eat healthy. For so long I thought I could never lose weight, because I thought it would take so much time to cook healthy foods. I thought I would have to cook six times a day—not true.

It's actually way faster to cook healthy food, because so little needs to change in order to eat it. The processed food in cans and frozen packages has to be thawed out and cooked in the oven to eat. Thawing pizza rolls on a baking sheet and putting them in the oven actually takes more time than throwing a piece of tilapia in a skillet. You can cook fish in a skillet in five minutes, chicken and vegetables in under ten minutes. Bottom line: you can enjoy the healthiest meal you can imagine in under ten minutes. When you first get started, it will take a little more time to learn new techniques, but once you expand your basic cooking skills, you'll use way less time than you think.

The key to making the most of your meal-prep time is *prep*aration. By taking one hour each week, you can make it convenient to eat healthy—and convenience is what we Americans are all about, right? I prep meals once a week because then I'm prepared when I go out, so I never have to think I don't have time to cook. On a Sunday, for example, I make all my chicken, lean ground turkey, vegetables, sweet potatoes—all of it, so I can choose healthy foods that are convenient, instead of swinging through drive-thru.

The truth is that most women have told themselves it will take too much time to eat healthy, even though they've never tried to do it. It's become an excuse to fail before they even get started. We have hundred of healthy recipes in the LadyBoss Lifestyle

Take long deep breathes. Short, quick breathing releases cortisol (the stress hormone) into your body, hindering weight loss.

Program to help women eat healthy without taking a lot of time. Most of them are really simple and take less than ten minutes to prepare. And when we talk about eating healthier snacks that require no prep time, we see it for what it is—an excuse. It doesn't take any more time to eat mixed nuts or to whip out some Nut Thins or Rice Thins.

Warning: You should *never, ever* get your meals from a drive-thru. There's almost nothing you can get from a drive-thru that will be good for you. If you're not willing to take five minutes to prepare a healthy lunch at home, why would you wait for five minutes or more in the drive-thru line to get unhealthy food?

Seriously, if you're not willing to pack a decent lunch then you're probably not serious about embracing a healthy lifestyle. Get up five minutes earlier and *make your freaking lunch!* Stop sleeping in. No more excuses. And no more *freaking* McDonald's!!

If you're going for a run, the jog.fm app will select songs for you to match your pace.

Big Fat Lie #10

You can lose weight quick with a magic pill or the perfect powder.

The Truth:

Good supplements support, not replace, good eating habits.

You can't eat McDonald's drive-thru food all day every day, then take a pill to lose weight and feel amazing. Nutritional supplements can be great and definitely have their place. But the truth is no matter what supplements you take, it isn't going to matter if you eat Krispy Kreme donuts and pizza every day.

Supplements are not replacements; there's no single pill or powder, no mysterious, magical break-through that will make you lose weight without changing your lifestyle. Anyone who tells you different is lying to you. When you're following a proven plan, supplements can definitely speed up the process. But you have to lead with your nutrition and supplement with the supplements.

So many women today lead with supplements, and supplement with nutrition. They eat *whatever* and hope the supplements will override poor nutrition. It doesn't work that way. You'll get into shape primarily by putting good nutrition into your body and working out really freaking hard. A supplement can help burn calories and boost your metabolism, but it can't replace the heart of the LadyBoss Formula: Fitness + Nutrition.

The key is to get the right kind of supplements. Ladies, a lot of supplements are made specifically for men, *so be careful*. Women have different hormones and unique tolerances. Make sure the supplements you take are designed with women in mind. That's why I started Lady-Boss Labs, so ladies could know that the supplements they use were created for them. One woman in the LadyBoss community told me she was trying to lose 60

You can't drink an empty water bottle! Little bottles run out fast. Best thing is to go to amazon.com and order a BIG ½ gallon jug to keep at home and/or the office.

pounds. I cheered her on and she sent me picture of what the guy at her local health food chain store sold her—a mass gainer! It was literally *designed* to help guys *gain* muscle. So many of those salespeople at chain stores know very little about the products they sell. They're just trying to push whatever is on sale at the time.

I have spent—I kid you not—tens of thousands of dollars on hundreds of nutritional supplements. When I attended fitness events, I would get tons of samples, and I tried almost all of them. That's how I know so many supplements out there are garbage. You can buy a huge bag of shake mix at the wholesale club stores that is nothing but crap—full of fillers and not formulated for you at all. Or you can invest in high-quality supplements designed to take your fitness and nutrition benefits to the next level. I invite you to check out LadyBossLabs.com for supplements I handcrafted for women just like you.

LadyBoss Success Story

Erika Sams, High Point, NC

I've been self-conscious about my weight since I was about 6 years old. However, through my late teens, I seemed to be able to eat whatever I wanted, and the weight would just fall off me. I wasn't slight or anything, but I was within the weight limits recommended for my height.

At 21, I had a beautiful son via cesarean delivery. The recovery was brutal. My health declined rapidly. I guess my unhealthy habits caught up to me, and between that and the development of a gluten allergy, I gained 90 pounds in less than a year. By the time I realized I couldn't eat gluten, I was too deep into the weight gain. I'd also never lived in a home with healthy eating or lifestyle habits, so I felt completely lost!

For the next 3 years I stumbled along, slowly losing about 15 pounds and gaining some "healthier" habits, but I had a long way to go and desperately needed some guidance.

When I first saw Kaelin's page, I thought, There is something different here; I can tell. Then, the day that the LadyBoss Movement was introduced with the lifetime membership, I had to jump! Workouts that were laid out, a menu that was already planned, and other woman going through the same thing to help hold me accountable—yes! But while I saw their results, would it really work that quickly for me?

OMG. Kaelin girl, if you get nothing else from this, just get this—thank you!

You have no idea how desperately I wanted and needed this. I'm gonna be real with you, and you can share this; I have nothing to hide. I take medicine for depression and anxiety. Following your menus, putting these healthy foods into my body, and giving it what it needs, of course I'm still taking my medicine too, but I am a THOUSAND times happier mentally because of taking care of myself physically! I'm losing weight; I've lost 11 pounds so far, and I've slimmed down noticeably. People around me are noticing my attitude change, and my confidence has boosted! It's to the point that it's actually motivating those around me to start working on getting healthier themselves!

Kaelin, I repeat—THANK YOU!! I'm seriously tearing up... I can't explain the huge difference this has made just in 3 months. I can't wait to see how it continues....

Chapter 10

Exercise Lies

Big Fat Lie #11

A gym membership will make you exercise.

The Truth:

Confidence and a proven game plan will empower you to exercise.

It happens every year, right after January 1st. Everybody signs up for a gym membership, thinking it will cause them to get healthy and lose weight. The exercise industry has sold the idea that losing weight and feeling great starts when you sign on the dotted line. We've connected a gym membership with the process of losing weight, but getting a gym membership won't make you embrace a healthier lifestyle. The truth is most people sign up and never go more than once or twice, if at all.

Planet Fitness is one of the largest gym chains in the country. The average Planet Fitness gym has about 6,000 members. Yet that same Planet Fitness only has capacity for 300 people. Why? They know that having a gym membership doesn't mean you're going to go to the gym. If it did, they'd have a gym twenty times the size they do. They know only 5% of people who have a gym membership actually use it.

What's the difference between those who go consistently and those who don't? Confidence and a proven game plan. The 5% who go consistently know what they are doing, and the rest of them don't. The first time I went to the gym, I wore a hoodie with the hood up so no one would see me. I literally walked in the gym, looked around at everyone else working out, and turned right around and walked back out. I had no clue what I was doing and felt so embarrassed. That's what a lot of people feel, maybe even you.

Having a gym membership isn't what gets people to work out

Mark your Calendar. Every day that you make it to the gym, make a large red "X" on your calendar to hold yourself accountable and stay motivated. You will feel compelled to keep the chain of X's going.

consistently. Having the confidence that comes from following a proven game plan—that's what matters. Confidence moves people to take the next action step. When you have a plan that's going to walk you through and make you feel comfortable, that shows you what to do where you can have confidence doing it, then you're going to do it. If not, you'll try to avoid the pain of embarrassment.

I think the same exact principle applies to food or any other part of healthy living. Having the gym membership, workout tool, diet plan, or product does not guarantee you know how to use it. It's not just the *what,* but the *how* that you need to succeed. Knowing how gives you the confidence to succeed and the knowledge of how to schedule it into your life.

For example, in the LadyBoss Lifestyle Program we provide a three-day, five-day and a seven-day training calendar based on how many days you want to train. We don't just give you the list of exercises to do or the list of foods to eat. We give you the workout plan. We give you the recipes. We give you a video to show you *how* to do the workout and *how* to cook the recipe. If you bought new running shoes, but didn't know how to tie them, you'd never run. It's the same principle across the board when it comes to healthy living.

If you know *what* to do and *how* to do it, you're far more likely to go to the gym, eat healthy meals, and continue to become the AWESOME person you truly are.

Keep a pair of workout clothes and shoes in your trunk. So on days you don't have time to pack your bag or you forget, you won't have an excuse not to go!

Big Fat Lie #12

Weight training is only for men and will make you big and bulky.

The Truth:

Building muscle helps you get rid of cellulite, burn calories and keep off the fat.

Building lean muscle is what gives you that toned, fit physique you really want. But a lot of women have bought into the lie that working with weights is only for men. They've been told weights will make them look bulky, so they should just stick to running or going to Zumba, cardio, and spin classes.

In fact, for some reason, women think *muscle* equals *masculinity*. It's just not true. Women who bulk up like men don't do that naturally. Trust me, I've been on the inside of the body-building industry. You've probably seen pictures of women who bulked up and look like freaking men with arms the size of my thighs! That is not going to happen to you if you touch a dumbbell. The truth that no one wants to talk about is those women are taking stuff to make them look that way. It's not going to happen otherwise.

It's not possible for women to naturally put on that type of muscle mass, because we don't have the testosterone in our bodies to create it. We have estrogen, which is sort of a muscle growth blocker. That's why it's harder for women to build muscle than it is for men.

The answer is that toning up—or building muscle—gets rid of cellulite, burns calories for three days after your training session, and helps you lose weight and keep it off.

We've been told that toning up means just doing cardio. Not true. All cardio does is make you a smaller version of yourself. It doesn't tighten your body up. It doesn't build any lean muscle on your body for you to have that sexy, toned physique. When you only do cardio all the time, you just end up skinny-fat.

I call them cardio-bunnies, women who think they're going to

Listen To Your Body! If something hurts then don't push it! Just remember there is a difference between the burn of effort and the pain of an injury.

get that sexy bikini body by doing cardio all the time. Doesn't happen. They end up with all the wiggles and jiggles in all the same places they used to have them, because they're not lifting weights. They're not building any muscle. Their body composition is not changing at all. They're becoming smaller but still have saddlebags and bat wings under their arms.

Getting fit is about more than doing cardio. What most women don't know is that they burn calories for up to three days after lifting weights. For example, when you get on an elliptical and do cardio for thirty minutes, you burn calories for that thirty minutes. Your body will continue to burn those calories for the next three hours. But when you weight train and you start building lean muscle, your body becomes a calorie-burning machine—literally. Your body will continue to burn calories for three days after that work out. Even when you aren't working out, you'll burn fat. When your body builds muscle, it uses energy and burns calories to sustain that muscle. Consequently, the more lean muscle you have, the more calories you burn *just by sitting there reading this book.*

Muscle itself doesn't weigh more than fat, like some people say. Five pounds is five pounds, whether it's made up feathers or bowling balls. Muscle is denser than fat, so it takes up less room in your body, but it requires more energy to sustain. If you work with weights three to five times a week, you keep your body in that metabolic state where it's constantly burning fat, especially that dreaded cellulite.

Cellulite is nothing more than fat pockets underneath your skin. Women always ask, *How do I get rid of this cellulite on the back of my legs? I've got cottage cheese legs and won't even wear shorts. I'm doing all this cardio, but none of my cellulite is going away. What*

Soak in an epsom salt bath to reduce muscle aches and pains.

are some creams to use? You don't need creams, and cardio won't get rid of cellulite.

What will work is building lean muscle in your legs while eating healthy. Eating healthy will lower your unhealthy fat intake. Toning up your muscles will get rid of fat pockets, craters where fat is stored because you're not getting sufficient circulation. As you lean down from eating healthy and building lean muscle, your cellulite will go away. That's what will give you those nice, lean legs all women want. Using weights helps you lose inches instead of just losing weight. It gives you that tight body you want.

I choose to carry a little more muscle than most women because of my championship figure, body-building efforts. I train every single day to maintain the muscle I have because I am in the top 3% of body types for women. But you don't have to do that much to look like the knock-out you truly are!

Lifting weights is NOT only for men. Leave that lie behind! If you want to look and feel great, drop those extra inches and finally get rid of that pesky cellulite, make weight training part of your normal workout routine. Members of the LadyBoss community have access to programs that make it easy to do. But you can check out my social media sites and learn enough to get you started on the right path. Soon you'll be burning fat, even when you're doing nothing—and looking great doing it!

Big Fat Lie #13

You can have it all without making sacrifices.

The Truth:

You can't enjoy the benefits unless you do the work.

Let me bring it home for you, ladies. Something's got to give. Everything you're sold by the weight-loss industry says you can have it all without making sacrifices. You don't have to give up anything; "just buy this program, take this pill, wrap special plastic around your belly and—*poof!* You'll lose weight and feel great." We've all heard the crazy claims. You can have great abs in five minutes a day. You can work all your muscle groups with a four-minute workout—blah, blah, blah. *We all know it's BS.*

The truth may not be popular, but you need to embrace it if you're ever going to experience real lifestyle transformation. You can't have all the benefits of doing the work without *actually* doing the work. If things are going to change for you, you will have to make sacrifices. You're going to have to sacrifice watching *The Bachelor, The Voice,* or your favorite shows every night. You're going to have to stop hiding behind the excuse of *I don't have the time.* You're going to have to realign your priorities to get to the gym and sacrifice some of your favorite foods. Pizza and ice cream will have to go—except for your weekly cheat meal, of course. You just can't keep eating that stuff every day and get the body you want. You'll have to make sacrifices to enjoy the weight-loss you dream about. You *can* do it, but it will cost you. Anybody who tells you differently is lying to you.

You can't keep doing what you're doing and expect to see different results. Your priorities have to change. Sitting on your sofa watching shows can't be your number-one priority. Scrolling through Facebook for an hour can't be your priority anymore. Underwater basket weaving—or whatever else you can imagine—can't be your priority anymore. Instead of being on Facebook, you can take that hour to do your

Walk on an incline treadmill after a leg workout to reduce soreness. This will help work out the lactic acid in your muscles.

weekly meal prep. Instead of sitting on the sofa, you can workout at the gym while you watch that show. You're going to have to do things differently.

If you want to achieve those dreams you wrote down earlier, it is *not* going to be easy. I'm just being real. But will it be worth it? Absolutely! You *can* achieve your new goals by setting new priorities. But then you have to act on those new priorities. None of the stuff you've read in this book will help you if you nod along with me then do nothing. None of the lies I've exposed or the truths I've shared will do you any good *unless* you do something about it.

You'll have to start something new, and you can't fill a full cup. You'll have to empty some out and make some sacrifices to create the room to grow and change. But it will be worth it when you have the energy each morning to get up and pursue your dreams. It will be worth it when you're able to keep up with your kids and grandkids decades from now. It will be worth it when you achieve that business success or get that promotion at work because you had the stamina and strength to get things done. There is no shortcut. There is no easy path. But you can do this! Whatever your dreams may be, it will be worth it when you see them come true.

LadyBoss Success Story

Jacqueline Borland, Reno, NV

Before LadyBoss, I was wandering the gym aimlessly, hoping I was hitting the right body parts, and crossing my fingers I would be sore the next day, because that meant it was working, right? I lost 30 pounds before I found Kaelin, and I decided to join because I was at a standstill. I couldn't get those inches to budge, and I couldn't get the scale to budge, and I had no clue why!

I came across Kaelin and saw her awesome results, and thought, If she can do it what's holding me up? So I took a leap of faith into the program. I now feel confident in the gym workouts on the open floor. Before I would only stick to the ladies' gym.

I feel confident in my clothes, and I can run around and play with my 4-year-old at the park, in fact, he gets tired before I do!

I'm steadily increasing the weights in my workouts, and even got to a point where I wasn't sore after leg day. I started eating more, which was a big challenge for me, and started incorporating carbs back into my diet. I'm still not where I want to be, but the most valuable thing being part of LadyBoss has given me is the ability to love myself every single day, and to value my gains no matter how small. Before, I was just seeing what I wasn't accomplishing.

I feel more muscular and less flabby everyday! And that is a huge victory for me! My results aren't staggering, or crazy dramatic, but I'm moving in the right direction again, and I wasn't sure

I could go farther than I had! I love this program and would recommend it to anyone that wants to gain confidence in themselves, both in and out of the gym.

Chapter 11

The LadyBoss Manifesto

If there's one thing I hope you get from this book, it's the simple but powerful TRUTH that I believe in YOU! You are capable of so many awesome things in life! Your story deserves to be one you LOVE to tell—and that brings joy to those you love.

I don't want you to continue in self-destructive habits or to settle for less than all you could be. You don't have to believe the LIES spread by the weight-loss industry to keep you paying for diet programs that don't work. Now that you know the TRUTHS you need to succeed, it's time for you to take action.

I want you to take charge of your life and choose your own destiny. No matter what has happened to you or how painful your life may feel right now, know that there is hope for a better tomorrow.

You are not alone. I have the privilege of connecting with tens of thousands of ladies just like you in the LadyBoss Movement. Being a LadyBoss has come to mean so much for so many that I thought I'd let our LadyBoss Manifesto speak for itself.

See if our Manifesto resonates with you:

A LadyBoss is the COURAGEOUS WOMAN inside of us who takes responsibility for where she's at. She isn't a victim of her circumstances. SHE DOESN'T MAKE EXCUSES or complain about what she can't change. She spends more energy DOING SOMETHING about it instead of telling everybody why she "can't".

A LadyBoss CAN HAVE IT ALL and do it all without having to compromise who she is or her integrity. A LadyBoss realizes that SHE SHINES the most when she is authentic and true to herself.

A LadyBoss isn't about just talk, but GETTING IT DONE. She recognizes that if she wants results and success, she has to PUT IN THE WORK. A LadyBoss doesn't aim to please others expectations, but rather aims to be THE BEST VERSION OF HERSELF she can be.

A LadyBoss doesn't listen to all the negative haters around her who are afraid she will succeed. A LadyBoss FOCUSES ON WHAT SHE WANTS instead of focusing on why she "can't".

A LadyBoss is a NO BS, TAKE ACTION, GET IT DONE, NO COMPROMISE WOMAN WHO VALUES HER INTEGRITY, CONFIDENCE, SELF-WORTH, AND DOESN'T CHANGE WHO SHE IS for anybody.

A LadyBoss is IN CONTROL of her destiny, her situation, her health, her body, and in turn, her life.

LadyBoss is a mentality that you choose to step into. It's your confident alter ego. It means putting aside all your doubts, all your fears, all of your excuses, and every reason why you think you can't do it.

BECAUSE YOU CAN DO IT!

If you're ready to take your life back, but know you need help, I invite you to connect with me and the tens of thousands of other ladies in the LadyBoss movement at LadyBoss.com.

You'll find all the help you need to take the journey to a healthier, happier YOU!

If this book has been a help to you, I'd love to hear about it. Post a message to me on any of the social media outlets listed at LadyBoss.com.

I SO look forward to hearing from YOU! Wherever your healthy lifestyle journey may lead, know that I'm cheering for YOU—because YOU ARE AWESOME!!

Start Your Journey at LadyBoss.com

More LadyBoss Success Stories

Morgan Deardorff, Auburn, WA

I became a lifetime LadyBoss, and all I can say is WOW! I may not have the most amazing weight-loss journey, but let me tell you what, it has definitely been a roller coaster!

From not eating enough, to eating too much, from only cardio, to using weights— it has definitely been a ride. Since starting this journey I have not only lost 5 pounds and 1% body fat but have also lost a jean size!

Along with that I have gained the most confidence I've ever had in my own skin. I don't feel the pressure to worry about what to meal prep nor dread eating salad or broccoli constantly. I walk into the gym with my head held high, and know I will crush my workout, because I know exactly what I'm going to do ahead of time.

The fit life is so much more than calories and being skinny. The LadyBoss program has given me the flexibility to live my life while getting in the best shape of my life! I have already come so far in 6 weeks and can't wait to see how much farther I can go! I get married next April and plan to blow everyone away! Thank you Kaelin for creating such an amazing and easy to follow program. You have changed my life for the better!

Meagan Wojtysiak, Bloomington, MN

Like so many other women, I tried MANY diets and plans. Some worked, and some didn't. Either way, I didn't get to where I wanted to be. I allowed setbacks to not only halt my progress, but also completely erase it—and then some. It was all so very discouraging.

When I found Kaelin's program, I was hesitant. First, I tried just doing the workouts and doing my own meal plan, based off of the recipes and guidelines. Then, I completely flipped it and started following the meal plan, but not working out a lot. I did this out of fear. Fear that if I would commit myself to the plan 100% that I would fail like the many times before.

It wasn't until recently that I had a "light bulb moment" from watching one of Kaelin's videos that caused me to center my focus around my #1 why: becoming confident again. As per Kaelin's advice, I use that #1 why EVERY second of EVERY day to motivate me. Because of this, I have been following both the meal plan and the workouts 100% FEARLESSLY, because I'm a LadyBoss now, and that's what we do!

So far, I have lost 10 lbs. and 21.5 inches overall. My progress has really taken off since I trusted in Kaelin and the LadyBoss Movement and I'm not looking back!!

Stephanie Willingham, Vero Beach, Florida

I've been on this roller coaster of a weight journey for years! I've tried so many different ways to lose weight, and would see some results, but then revert back to my old ways. This always made me gain back the weight and more! I've battled emotional eating and food addiction, not realizing these were my problems.

I've been following Kaelin for years. I sometimes looked into her posts or watched her videos, but nothing quite connected with me until I saw her LadyBoss Movement introduction. I loved the amount of helpful information and support from fellow LadyBosses! I went from making every excuse to not work out, justifying eating junk food, not wanting to start my journey to now loving my daily gym time, eagerness to prepare healthy meals and loving myself!

I don't know what would have happened to me if I didn't take that time to see what being a LadyBoss was about. Thank you Kaelin and fellow LadyBosses from the bottom of my heart!! We are all beautiful and strong women who deserve to live a happy, healthy life.

Amber Schmidt, Killdeer, North Dakota

Before LadyBoss, I was lost, struggling with which program to use, what supplements and vitamins to take, when do I take everything and when do I exercise?

Then I found LadyBoss on Facebook and thought, What the heck, I've done EVERYTHING else, why not this too?

Little did I know how much all the help and information that I got from this program would truly help. I like doing the workouts; I like the meal plans/grocery list; I like the website, but most of all, I get a huge kick and encouragement from the Facebook group.

I have lost 9 pounds plus a few inches too, and I couldn't be happier! I know it's not a lot of pounds, but to me it is HUGE! I have been on the fence of 200 pounds for 12 years, and to see me take my time and not worry about the pounds, but work on eating better and keeping active— it feels so stinking good to finally say I am in striking distance of seeing the scale hit 189 soon!

I can't say it enough— thank you, and GOD Bless!

Kaylenn Gosman, Louisville, KY

I have always been the "fat" friend. All of my friends in high school were smaller than me; all my friends in college were smaller than me, and all my friends now that I work with are smaller than me.

I have tried it all, from crash diets, diet pills, detox teas, weight-loss shakes— you name it, and I've done it. But those were all temporary for me. I'd be on it strong for a week and then drop it because I wasn't seeing results.

One day I was laying in bed, upset about my weight— which was an everyday thing—and saw Kaelin had posted a live feed. I had never heard of her or her progress or program before; one of my friends had shared it. So I watched her 45 minute feed and ended up buying the lifetime deal with LadyBoss.

With this program I feel like a completely different person. I'm down 16 pounds so far and can't wait to see how far it will take me. I was obsessed with the scale but have since gotten rid of it and gone off of progress pictures, measurements, and the feel of my clothes.

Have I fallen off the wagon in this journey? Yes, but I get right back on, because I know this is something that works, and it's not temporary. If I can work 12-hour night shifts as an ICU RN and do this program, anybody can. I will never forget the day I randomly met Kaelin in Louisville at the gym and the encouragement she gave me! She cares about her LadyBosses and their progress! I love this lifetime program!!!

CPSIA information can be obtained
at www.ICGtesting.com
Printed in the USA
LVOW10s0412300317
528996LV00032BA/911/P